D1579932

Kiss & MaKe uP

Praise for 'Kiss and Make Up'

'Carl's brave, honest and hugely entertaining story transported me right back to the eighties when we all felt anything was possible with a bit of glitter, lots of attitude and Grace Jones playing full blast. I laughed and cried and above all could not stop turning the pages. A cracking read and I want to hear more from this talented writer.'

Lorraine Kelly – TV presenter

'A great ride. Raw, messy, sometimes a laugh, sometimes a heartbreaker, usually wildly over-dressed, this first-person tale of survival is a bit like the pop-haunted decades it whirls us back into – years when being a young queer took a lot of nerve as well as a lot of eyeliner.'

Neil Bartlett – playwright, director, performer and writer

'Carl Stanley is a natural born writer. Whatever else he is, I couldn't possibly comment. You'll just have to read his highly entertaining memoir and find out for yourself!'

Paul Burston – author and founder of 'Polari' literary salon

'Carl's turn of phrase paints a very unique picture of the '80s – heavy with intrigue, experimentation, and finally revelation!'

Princess Julia – Culture Correspondent at iD magazine

'Carl sets his own soundtrack to this vivid and colourful book about a sexually confused teenager growing up in the '80s. I'm thrilled to have been a part of that soundtrack and an inspiration for this wonderful book that captures the time perfectly — a time when the genders became blurred by many of the major stars. Sexual ambiguity, make-up and fashion all played a part to give teenagers of the time more freedom for their sexual expression than ever before. The '80s was a wonderful, horrible, confused time, and young gay teenagers were able to have a first taste of freedom despite the conservative moral attitudes of crusades that marred the era.'

Marc Almond — singer and author

'How thrilling it is to have been part of Carl's colourful life! The '80s was a time of exploration, gratification and living the dream, a dream that at times could be a nightmare, other times paradise. Every generation has 'the dream': there was the '60s, the '70s then the '80s! The '80s allowed gender confusion, in fact it welcomed it, and the decade allowed us all to love whomever we wanted to love as we all fought bigoted attitudes with wit and aplomb. Even so, these journeys are not always easy, and Carl's eloquent, witty and wicked writing is a wonderful statement to the glory of this decade.'

Toyah Willcox — singer, actress and author

Kiss & MaKe uP

by

Carl Stanley

Ignite BooKs
2015

ISBN: 978-0-9932044-1-8

Typeset by Steve at Ignite.
www.ignitebooks.co.uk

Printed and bound in the UK
by CPI Group (UK) Ltd
Croydon. CR0 4YY.

Dedicated to Mom, to Marc, and to all those who,
for better or for worse,
left their marks.

'When you were afraid I was there by your side
when you were alone I was your place to hide
but always in your mind you were some place far away
you were someone else I didn't really know at all.'

'Scar' Marc Almond

Chapters

1

'To those who will survive...'

'*Moments of Pleasure*' Kate Bush

November 26th, 2005.

"So who are you then?" asked Great-uncle George as I defied gusty drizzle and finally struck a match, determined to enjoy what – unless she was late – would be my final fag 'til after the service. Inhaling at leisure, I held the smoke then slowly breathed my name.

"Carl."

"No! I'd never've recognised you! Last time I saw you, you were wearing rouge an' lipstick an' a frock, and you had black hair an' you were really mardy!" he laughed. Now, in my mid-thirties, grown into my looks and at one with being ginger, I could smile at that cross-dressed teenage ego of yesteryear.

"Ooh, and when you were little you made your mom's life hell," he went on.

Bet she never told you she made my childhood hell, I thought, and shuddered at the memory, as George acknowledged Dad who'd come out to preach about the perils of smoking – the fiscal, not the physical.

Punctual for once, Nan pulled up tailed by two cars – three of her grandsons, her three kids and two of their spouses stepping into the mizzle in a muddle of umbrellas. Dad scurried back inside the church – long past its prime, in desperate need of some TLC which the unfilled collection plates of a dwindling Anglican congregation wouldn't bestow – and I darted towards the cortege to greet my aunts, uncles, cousins, mother and brother. Mom's immense cupola of a hat impeded anything closer than a distant hug, but had she been hatless it would've been the same; plus, relations between us had been more strained than ever lately, since she'd read the first draft of my version of our story. She looked much younger than sixty-whatever-she'd-admit-to. I pondered the flashy floral tributes: 'MOM' definitely wasn't Mom's want when such schmaltz wasn't her style, just as the one spelling 'NAN' hadn't come from me or Aidan. We three weren't doing the weepy thing either. Not that we were any less sad than anyone else, just more philosophical: Alzheimer's had taken our well-groomed dearly beloved many moons before death took the shabby stranger she'd become …

The stained glass Christ gazing down on Nan's casket had borne witness to her whole life: her christening, her wedding, the christenings of her four children, and the memorial services of her husband and youngest son. After the vicar had praised Winnie's Christian spirit and talked of her fame within the parish of St. Matthew's, Smethwick, a breadline district on the outskirts of Birmingham, she summoned Janet. My mom stood in front of the altar where she'd been married too, paid homage to an adored affectionate grandmother, and then touched upon their sometimes tense relationship, a few pews creaking as the discomfited shifted in their seats. She was a pro at detaching her public and private selves – one a self-possessed go-getter, the other a minefield – and she almost made it through before breaking. At once I saw an orphaned child, crying, wracked by unresolved pain. Reliving all those times when I'd wished her dead and she'd probably wished I'd never existed, I began to cry too. It didn't have to be too late for us, the living, but the ball was in her court now...

2

'It's a mystery to me...'

'It's A Mystery' Toyah

February 24th, 1981.

It's a tremendous change for someone of, if I may say, nineteen to make, the reporter suggested to Lady Di.

Janet had been nineteen when she'd married, too. It'd be their twentieth wedding anniversary this August, and while tradition might dictate the gifts should be of china, frustration might cause her to hurl another china plate at John instead...

"Pah, she doesn't know what she's letting herself in for! It'll be a damned sight easier for her than it is for me though. She won't have to cook an' clean an' run herself ragged picking up after three ingrates like I do," griped Mom, although that wasn't strictly true. Because not only had she employed a cleaner for years, she'd also gone into semi-retirement last summer...

Over dinner in 1980 she'd pronounced in a fit of pique, "Well if you lot can do as you flippin' well please, so can I! You're not cripples, there's gonna be big changes around here!"

Before she'd even finished eating she'd drawn up house-rules, reading aloud as she wrote:

1. I WILL ONLY WASH WHAT'S PUT IN THE LAUNDRY BASKET. SMELLY SOCKS DON'T WALK DOWNSTAIRS BY THEMSELVES
2. I REFUSE TO IRON FIFTEEN SHIRTS A WEEK SO LEARN TO DO IT YOURSELVES
3. I WILL ONLY COOK WHEN IT SUITS ME BUT I'LL STOCK THE FREEZER SO YOU CAN FEND FOR YOURSELVES ON MY DAYS OFF
4. JOHN WILL COOK DINNER EVERY SATURDAY, NO EXCUSES

"And they're effective from now which'll give you chance to get used to how it'll be when I'm in hospital having my hysterectomy."

"What's a hysterectomy?" I'd asked.

"Something I should've had twelve years ago," had been her flippant comeback as she'd pinned her commandments to the cork noticeboard.

Later, I'd trawled through the 'H's in my *Collins Gem*: **hysterectomy** *n*. the surgical removal of the womb.

Hang on a mo', if I'm eleven an' it takes nine months to have a baby... I'd thought.

Frosty and irascible, she'd never been especially likeable, but that comment had been the cherry on the icing of a cake of dislike that started two Christmases earlier in 1978 when the *Girl's World* I'd written Santa for wasn't under the tree. I'd hunted high-and-low lest he'd hidden it elsewhere, and she got so annoyed with me badgering her about where else could it be that she said, 'Nowhere because he isn't real.' I should've known really. She'd never have allowed anyone in Wellington

17

boots to step on her Axminster, not even a saint. One faith insensitively crushed, the next November she'd crushed another…

Soon after cancer had rotted Uncle Kevin – nine years my senior and my hero; so into Bowie he'd even had an *Aladdin Sane* mullet; a self-confessed 'vinyl junkie' with an eclectic record collection of Glam, Disco, Punk, Kate Bush and every genre in between – she'd announced, "We're not going to church again. God doesn't exist or she wouldn't have let my brother die."

"Will I have to leave school as well?" I'd asked.

"Don't ask stupid questions!"

"It's not stupid, my school's Church of England, we have to say prayers everyday an' go to church every Fri – "

"You're staying there, it's the top school in the area, just stop praying!"

"But what if there is a God? Won't he be angry?"

"Listen, if there is a God and I've angered *HER* by telling you *SHE* doesn't exist an' not taking you out of a religious school, I'm prepared to sacrifice your redemption for the sake of your education…and in any case, you won't be going to Heaven 'cause you weren't christened. Now stop the stupid questions unless you want what for!"

No Father Christmas, no Heavenly Father, possibly hell-bound, all I'd had left to hold onto was *me* but then she'd tried to crush that too…

Early that same year when Mom had gone into semi-retirement, I'd been captivated by a photo in *Smash Hits* of some fantastical creatures posing deadpan in a London night-club called The Blitz. With exotic aliases like Steve Strange and Princess Julia, collectively referred to as Blitz Kids or New

Romantics, citing David Bowie as their inspiration, I knew Uncle Kevin would've loved them, God rest his soul. For weeks I'd been obsessing about what type of New Romantic I'd make-up to be, and that half-term, while Mom was out shirking motherhood elsewhere, I'd raided her vast arsenal…

One hour later, half my face was laminated in gold, I had an oversized pink pout outlined in turquoise, eyes scarlet squares and a thin blue mono-brow drawn across the middle of a silver forehead, and I was posturing in my bedroom mirror to *'Boys Keep Swinging'* – which was amongst the records I'd inherited from Uncle Kevin. The music had been blaring so loud that even with bionic hearing I wouldn't have heard her enter…

"WHAT THE HECK ARE YOU DOING?!"
Gobsmacked, I stuttered "I… I… I…. I…"
"I'm not surprised you're stuck for words! Scrub that muck off, you look like a bloomin' clown!" ordered Mom – who was only marginally less coloured-in than me – as she trailed me to the bathroom because she still had plenty to say…
"And what were you thinking, putting lipstick 'round your eyes? It'll make you blind! Right, it's high time you start behaving like a normal eleven-year-old boy. Normal boys don't play with Barbies and dolls houses, they don't suck their thumbs and they certainly don't wear make-up! Enough is enough! Boys Brigade'll knock the sissy outta you *and* it'll get you out of my hair one night a week as well! Car, *now!* Unless you want what for…"

She'd flown two red lights, skidding to a halt outside the community centre, dragging me into a hall ripe with that same rubber odour as those hated gym mats at school.

"Can I help you, madam?" trilled the Company Leader, a John Inman impersonator who wasn't the sort of man any sane mother would entrust with butching-up her effeminate son.

"Yes. Carl wants to join Boys Brigade," Mom fibbed.

He'd looked me over, his beady stare landing on my face which – so great was Mom's urgency to get me there that she couldn't wait for me to wash properly – still twinkled with glitter.

"I'm very sorry madam, there's no space for *him* here," he'd sniffed haughtily, rolling his head and arching a brow. "Try Scouts."

But rather than risk Group Scout Leader's refusal too, Mom abandoned half-measures and enrolled me to sit the entrance exam to Aidan's school – a centuries-old, all-boys establishment which erased individuality with encyclopaedic rules *(Hair must be worn 1" above collar height; Ties must be worn in a 1¾" Windsor knot; Shoes must be…)*, and which prided itself on manufacturing alpha males through a programme of sports-sports-and-more-sports and its own Cadet Corps, all in return for exorbitant fees. Recoiling in horror at the prospect of all that rugby-rugby-and-more-rugby and military manoeuvring which my brother Aidan revelled in, and the prospect of zero girls, I'd begged "No, *pleeease,* I wanna go to the same seniors as Smuffle!"

"Who the hell's Smuffle?" Mom had asked.

Smuffle had been my long-time partner-in-crime.

Back in 1977, one playtime Sandra-as-then-was had proposed "We need funny nicknames", and as I'd taken to fantasizing being anybody but me – ideally some wealthy foreigner, which was why I'd lie

I'm French; my dad's a zillionaire – I'd agreed.

"What about Ethel an' Eddie?" she'd suggested.

"Hm, dunno, s'not that funny, how about Uffle an' Uddie?"

Hemming and hawing, only half-sold because surely she could invent something funnier, after much head-scratching, she'd exclaimed "I'VE GOT IT! Ya know the Smurfs? Let's put 'sm' in front an' call ourselves Smuffle an' Smuddie!"

"And let's put 'sm' in front of every word we say an' make our own language an' only speak to each other in it" I'd elaborated.

"Smrilliant!" she'd smirked. Inspired by the impending Silver Jubilee we'd stood on a bench and proclaimed

"SMALL SMOU SMEASANTS SMUST SMALL SMUS 'SMYOUR SMAJESTY' SMOR SME SMON'T SMALK SMO SMOU, SMUT SMOU SMUSTN'T SMALK SMOO SMUS SMIN SMOUR SMANGUAGE!"

Our declaration of the rights or lack thereof of peasants had gone down such a storm with our classmates that whenever we were separated for disrupting lessons, they'd willingly chance teacher's wrath to relay our royal dispatches from desk-to-desk. We enjoyed three years without a whiff of revolt, with curtseys and bows everywhere we'd go. It was the closest I'd get to being true royalty; I'd been in love with Princess Anne, and my plan had been to marry her until she put the kibosh on it by marrying Captain Mark Phillips when I was four…

Mom hadn't met Smuffle; in all those years I'd never once invited her 'round as I hadn't wanted to expose her to Mommie Dearest.

"Oh, I don't wanna know who this *Smuffle* is! You're sitting it and that's that…and you're intelligent enough to pass so you

WILL pass, unless you want what for," she menaced. Five years of public school torture or five seconds of hers, it'd been a no-brainer.

At the end of a monotonous morning examining row-upon-row of middle-aged juniors – all regimentally dull, ties *just so* and hair *just so* and they weren't even pupils yet, confirmation that this young abiders' institution definitely wasn't for me with my shoulder-length Purdy pageboy hairdo – secure I'd done my absolute worst I'd handed in my entry to comp then skulked out, loins girded for Mom's bottom-stinging 'what for'…

That teatime, Dad, playing devil's advocate, had said "Think of the thousands we'll save, Jan…and he did say he didn't wanna go to Solihull School, love."

"DON'T *'LOVE'* ME! You're *NO* bloody support," she'd played her broken record; "Why the hell does everything revolve 'round what you three want? Well if you lot can do as you flippin' well please…" and up had gone those house-rules, Mom-in-war-mode-thus-not-to-be-opposed appending, "And John, take him for a haircut…an' I don't mean a trim! Christ, if he wore a skirt people would think he was a girl!"

With Dad settled in the barber's chair, I'd distracted myself from Mom's barbaric sentence by thumbing the porno mags Georgiou thoughtfully provided for his customers' pleasure. Page after page of knockers: ones like Space Hoppers or droopier than beanbags, some with nipples like fried eggs; a fanny that reminded me of those Venus Flytraps I'd seen at the Botanical Gardens and no less terrifying for being toothless, a half-page close-up of red-taloned fingers stretching a hairless one wide apart to show off innards, not dissimilar to Dr

22

Spock's ears only rawer and soggier; and yuckier still a full-page close-up of it swallowing a pearl necklace and oozing goo at the same time. Then out of the blue, under the banner *'One for the Ladies'* leapt an athletic youth sporting naught but a cocky grin, his half-mast chopper a sight for sore eyes after countless icky cracks. Doing what any virtuous boy would, I'd freed him from vagina hell...

"Somethin' for the weekend, sir?" Georgiou had winked, brushing down Dad's neck.

"No, I'm fine thanks. Jan was sterilized after we had him...did I tell you she's goin' in to have a hysterectomy?" Dad had blathered, embellishing his 'no' with a tad too much information; "C'mon Caroline, over you come, let George do his job, no tantrums."

Pocketing *'One for the Ladies'*, feeling harder and manlier than ever, I shuffled across hand-in-pocket, and Georgiou could have turned me into Kojak for all I cared...

The second we'd got home I'd shot up the stairs two at a time, locked myself in the bathroom and unfolded *'One for the Ladies'*. Well into my stroke, there'd been a brusque *rat-a-tat-tat*.

"SHOW ME YOUR HAIR, SUNSHINE! HURRY UP, YOU'VE BEEN IN THERE AGES, IT'LL MAKE YOU BLIND!"

"I HAVEN'T TOUCHED YOUR MAKE-UP," I'd panted truthfully, my nuts tingling tighter than ten toes in a sock like they might burst...

"I'M NOT TALKING ABOUT MAKE-UP!"

Perverting the truth, I'd puffed, "CAN'T I EVEN POOH IN PEACE?" – visualising anything to reverse the surging splurge: Nan's surgical stockings, the Queen Mother's yellow teeth, fannies, *her*...

"DON'T MAKE A MESS, SON!"
Too late!

Emptying a canister of *Ainwick* to uphold my lie that I'd been poohing, opening the door warily, Mom had almost fallen in on top of me – lamely acting-out she was busting to wee despite there being a downstairs lav, guiltlessly lying regardless of always flipping her lid whenever she'd suspect I had, no mention of the mannish crop she'd been so desperate to see, an almost instant flush upholding her lie that she'd been peeing.

But here we were, watching telly on 24th February, 1981, and seeing as neither months of frequent lipstick around my eyes nor compulsive masturbation had caused blindness I believed jack shit Mom said these days...

"Another scrounger we'll have to support...the government should confiscate all their money...*our* money...except some to buy council houses on the right-to-buy scheme... and they should be made to work for a bloody living like everybody else," grumbled Mom, who for all her republican bollocks had nevertheless chosen a regal rosewood-panelled front door whose stately brass fittings she'd religiously buff. 'It's like the entrance to Versailles,' my clarinet teacher had said.

"Shush, *mother!*"
"Don't *shush* me, it's my television!"

And, I suppose, in love? prompted the reporter.
Of course, Lady Di simpered, affecting indignation – her fiancé adding
Whatever 'in love' means...it's your own interpretation.
I'd been in love with '*One for the Ladies*' 'til we were torn

apart two weeks prior by an outraged Mom who'd given me 'what for'. I was hopelessly in love with dramatic cosmetics, and the way they could disguise my genetics to help stop me looking so much like *her*. I was also in love with Toyah – musically, for her Satsuma-colour mop, for riling tyrannical Mom who'd branded her a pleb for saying 'shit' on telly – and in spite of my being an ardent royalist, far more electrifying than the Royal betrothal was today's other historic event: with five flop singles under her belt, Toyah's sixth had crashed the Top 40, straight in at No.26.

Well, it obviously means...er...obviously two very happy people, the reporter enlightened Prince Charles.

"Big-eared plonker..."

"Shut up will you, *mother!*"

"Don't you dare take that tone with me *sunshine* or you'll get what for!"

Having her reproductive organs ripped out may have calmed her down somewhat, but 'what for' still meant the cane. I think 'what for' had first appeared in the wake of Granddad's death – six or so years earlier when I was six – although that period was a bit of a blur, a nightmare that family consciousness chose to let sleep. While its appearance was usually deterrent enough not to backchat – or sufficient stimulus to fess up to whatever felony we'd been accused of, whether culpable or not – she'd often follow through with a thwack anyway. She could insist they were only slight taps 'til her face turned cobalt, but slight taps wouldn't have necessitated drastic action. Last week, after one 'slight tap' too many, in Mom's absence Aidan and I had taken possession of that stick that was weightless as air but stung like hell... sprinting to a blind spot by the pond where we'd be unseen should she unexpectedly return...having to bend her damned scourge back on itself before it would snap, then again, then again, maniacally splintering the quarters under heel, sweeping them into the water and burying them under duckweed... finally free...pledging that if she replaced it we'd smash that one too.

"And as for her an' her *Shy Di* routine, she's a car crash waiting to happen..."

"For Chrissake, *mother,* either shut up or go away," I cheeked with the cockiness of one who couldn't be caned, and off she went, ransacking the cloakroom only to reappear empty-handed.

"Are you looking for something?" I pushed, interested to hear what punishment she'd mete.

"RIGHT, ROOM! NOW! AND DON'T EVEN *THINK* ABOUT PLAYIN' YOUR MUSIC OR I'LL CONFISCATE YER STEREO *AND* STOP YOUR ALLOWANCE!"

When she was extremely furious like she was now, her pitch rose a thousand decibels and fifty octaves. The surgeon would've done us — and dogs the universe over — a favour if he'd ripped out her vocal chords too. She might believe she'd found new means to hit where it hurt, but God clearly detested her as much as I did or He wouldn't have invented headphones...

'The big quethtion mark in hithtory,' lisped Toyah.

My big questions were why Mom and Dad were together when their love wasn't like Chas and Di's, why they'd had us when they didn't love us. In our house 'love' was just four-letter damage limitation Dad would say to pre-empt or pacify Mom's anger, a word they'd only ever squander on us in birthday or Christmas cards. *Whatever love is* – and it wasn't the fivers our hands-off Dad threw our way or her heavy hands-on approach – *it's a mystery to me...*

3

'A fold in an eyelid brushed with fear...'

'The Sound of the Crowd' Human League

My new best mate and I had been kept behind after Maths for collaging our books in pictures of Toyah clipped from magazines. Miss Downs – reaching in the cupboard behind her desk for a roll of brown paper – stating the obvious, asked, "So, are you two Toyah fans?"

Rich and I pulled mong faces...

Spinning around, she continued, "Her parents are my neighbours. Bring a couple of things in and I'll leave them with Mr and Mrs Willcox for her to sign."

Once we'd winched up our jaws and were done brown-wrapping Toyah, we swore we'd never again say *Downs must be a lezza* just because she bore an uncanny resemblance to Billie Jean King, or call her *Downs Syndrome*, or make spaz faces at her back. We even did our homework at lunchtime in order to free up precious time that night to discuss which of the scores of artefacts – bought with pocket money and earnings from our early morning paper rounds – we'd bring in next day...

That morning we went in laden with thirty record sleeves

and an entire rainforest of fanzines and posters between us. Weeks later Miss Downs struggled back in with everything. Unsigned...

"Toyah's on tour abroad, she won't be visiting them in the near future," she relayed all too gaily, as we gathered up our stuff. She rummaged in her briefcase, ignoring our disappointment. *Vile lezza*, I thought...

"But they gave me these."

She produced two tickets to Toyah's Birmingham show.

"Now don't thank me, just promise you'll work harder, okay?"

"Yes Miss," we paid lip service.

I told Rich an image overhaul would be essential or we'd look a proper pair of dorks in our velour zip-up tops and Farahs. We had to look cool at our first concert.

"What should we wear then?" he asked.

Ideally I knew it would be something Steve Strange-ish or like Bowie in the *'Ashes to Ashes'* video, but as far as I was aware nowhere in Solihull sold outfits like theirs, so I suggested we opt for something more DuranDuran instead: pixie boots, frilly shirts, trendy trousers, glittery scarves, make-up...

"S'pose wearin' pixie boots an' trousers like John Taylor's is alright but we ain't wearin' the rest or people'll think we're puffs," scoffed Rich.

He'd first said the 'p' word during our first exchange. Filing out of French one day, I'd noticed he had 'Toyah' on his rucksack.

"Hey, Rich, how long have you been into Toyah?" I'd asked, curious as to how this vital info had escaped me 'til then.

"Er, since I saw that documentary last December, d'ya see it?"

Yes, I had. That sixty minute profile on the Brummie-born pint-size Punkette, the self-appointed 'voithe of dithcontented youth', was what'd switched me on to her too.

"Fuckin' bostin weren't it? I got 'er first three albums last Christmas, bought *Anthem* the day it come out," he'd gone on.

"Me too," I'd gushed, indicating their four titles nestled amongst 'Soft Cell' and 'Visage' and every pop star worth their weight in eyeliner on a holdall roll-call I added to each week as another NewRo band catapulted their way to Top Ten fame.

"Yeah, I seen those...that '*Tainted Love*' singer's a right puff...weren't sure whether I should talk to ya tho' cuz some o' the lads reckon *you're* a puff."

"Why?" I'd gasped, thinking I'd done a brilliant job of hiding it. After all, it had been plain from day one that I'd have to...

That very first morning, drawn into an unruly rabble squashing itself through an entry built for single file in a century when children should be seen and not heard, making my way inside unscathed but dishevelled, I stopped to tuck my shirt in when "GIMME ME BACK MY CURLY WURLY YOU FUCKIN' WANKER!" bruised the riotous hubbub. I was shoved aside by some boy shouting "OUT MY FUCKIN' WAY, YA PUFF!" as he hurtled down the corridor holding his ill-gotten gain aloft like an Olympic torch. Then the victim barged past, pursuing him as speedily as her hobble skirt would allow, shouting at me "WATCH WHERE YOU'RE GOIN' YA PUFF!" Slipping on the granite she went arse-over-tit, splitting a seam as she fell, effing'n'blinding. Two tight-skirted girls helped her up, indelicately cussing after him on her behalf, and I concluded that the tighter the skirt, the commoner the girl. Returning to gloat, the sweetie thief flashed a gooey gobful and gunned "FUCKIN' SLAGS!"

Slags were clearly the kind of gals this establishment produced, as the summer hols just gone I'd read in *The Solihull News* that Mandy Rice-Davies – the call-girl who'd bedded Lords embroiled in The Profumo Affair, then named them under oath and helped topple an entire government, whose memoirs had just been published – was an ex-pupil; and it wasn't incomprehensible that graffiti claiming *'UR MOM GIVES BJS 4 5P'* and *'YOUR MOM OWS R DOG FOCK MONEY'* was dedicated to the maternal alumni of today's hobble-skirted girls...

The Curly Wurly thief's tie was tied in a fat knot; the rougher the boys the fatter their knots it seemed, substantiated when two gangs of yobs with particularly fat knots began volleying expletives, threatening to settle last year's old scores before the school-bell had even rung-in this one. Right away I retied mine super-skinny. As I combed my locks, which Mom had let grow long again, the sparring Fat Knots forgot their differences to turn as one and spout "PUFFTA!"

Suddenly, five-foot-ten of virility, the spit of gold medal swimmer David Wilkie appeared – sky blue trackies taut across his tackle which was double the dimensions of Mom's roll-on *MUM*, its explicit outline filed under *wank fodder* – and bellowed, "KNOCK IT OFF LADS, OR IT'LL BE A HUNDRED LAPS OF THE SOCCER PITCH!"

Dunno how they can tell I thought, swaggering John Wayne-style into the hall where we were being assigned to our forms...

"Miss, ya know it says Mrs Daniels is takin' us fer English?" asked one Fat Knot innocently as we copied our timetables.

Mrs Moore, prim as a doily, peered over her pince-nez spectacles...

"Is *she* that Mrs Daniels our bruvver told us was caught ridin' a fifth year she tied to a chair?"

That was adequate ammo to spark a crotch-grabbing mass debate over who was best equipped to get stuck into English next – soft-spoken Mrs Moore's feeble stab at restoring order drowned-out by the Fat Knots banging their desk tops in lieu of Mrs Daniels. Wilkie-lookalike Mr Pearce didn't merit a murmur, although I'd stake *'One for the Ladies'* on it that Alan – legs crossed, pout-lipped, tie as thin as mine and the one boy besides me not participating in the hullabaloo – would be gawking at it in PE too. Alan wasn't someone I'd want to associate with though: he had specs and acne and his attaché case wasn't emblazoned with 'Hazel O'Connor' or 'Gary Numan' or any pop star at all. Actually, from the coarse marker-penned logos I *could* decipher around me, no boys shared my tastes. Those who were musos were either Heavy Metal 'ead-bangers or well-'ard Ska nuts. Since it was obvious that only a complete Joey with a death-wish would betray himself as *a puff*, I'd joined in the desk-top-banging and tried to sustain that macho swagger and not perv at Mr Pearce's rounders bat or scream each time balls flew my way.

"Cuz you only hang out with Em an' Helen. An' there's that stuff Abi keeps sayin' 'bout you playin' with dolls," illuminated Rich when first we spoke.

She'd spread *that* at Infants' as well, thanks to a Judas playmate's loose lips, and separate Juniors' hadn't wiped it from her memory...

"Abi's a liar! And I hang out with Helen an' Em because I fancy them," I lied.

Rich, satisfied I wasn't a puff, proposed "Ya wanna be

mates then? Cuz we oughta be, both bein' into Toyah."

A gazillion per cent positive there'd be no outing myself in a fit of unbridled passion – unless the chubby carrot-top were to morph without warning into that spunky wan skinnymalink with the inky Mohican, Matthew Ashman, BowWowWow's guitarist – I spat on my palm like lads did, offered it Rich, we shook, and we'd been inseparable ever since. For appearances' sake I'd even tongued girls at the roller-disco…

Like Smuffle before him, I never invited Rich 'round either. And so what if Rich's inelegant jumble of a lounge stank of fags and Old English sheepdog? It was homelier than our sterile show home. His mom would insist *Make yourself comfy, put your feet up* – deemed an offence against champagne dralon chez moi which would invoke a diatribe along the lines of *Get yer stinky socks off my sofa, you'll wear it out; it'll have to last us long after you're gone!* Mrs B would supply endless sweet teas and bickies which Mom wouldn't have done for a comatose hypoglycaemic, and what's more, Mrs B would welcome me night-after-night whereas Mom would groan *You're back* every time I returned as if she hoped that when I'd left the house earlier it'd been for good even though I barely had enough pubes to plait.

So here Rich and I were, deliberating our concert clothes. Deaf to my argument that nobody could ever accuse lady-killers DuranDuran of being nancies, Rich could limit himself to new boots and trousers if he liked but I craved the whole nine yards if Mom would fork out for them. All I'd have to do was catch her in the right mood, which tended to be breakfasts the morning after her and Dad's headboard had banged long and steadily against the wall in the witching hour. Shopping that Saturday, freshly-serviced Mom was in such a generous mood that although she'd already spent-spent-spent on navy suede pixie boots, frothy white blouse and peacock-blue drainpipes, when we couldn't find an appropriately Duranish scarf, Stepford Mom beamed, "You can have my stripy gold one, you've always loved it, it's very DuranDuran."

I'd still need make-up though, but however liberal she was being today, however au fait she was with the *'Girls On Film'* look I was after, I knew from her overreaction when she caught me smeared in hers, that *that* request would be pushing it…and the skinhead haircut she'd make me have as punishment wasn't at all Simon Le Bon… No, I thought, with this month's allowance already gone on Toyah's brand-new LP *'The Changeling'*, it would be wiser to wait a fortnight for next month's allowance and buy my make-up on my own. But – flicking through Jo's *Jackie* in German when I should've been conjugating verbs – I found that the *voithe of dithcontented youth* who had launched her own cosmetics line was now *benefactreth to intholvent youth* too: **'FREE MAKE-UP FROM TOYAH!***' cried the headline.

"Oi, Rich, look! We've gotta send away for some!" I wriggled, close to wetting myself.
"Yeah, but we ain't gonna use it, it's fer our Toyah collections, right?" he checked charily.
Nodding dishonestly, reading the small print *'*simply mail us the coupon and a 29p stamp P&P to claim yours. Limited offer while stocks last'*, I said "Let's ask Jo an' Helen for their coupons an' run to the Post Office at lunchtime an' spend our dinner money on stamps an' envelopes in case they run out!"

The small print had also stated *'Please allow 21-28 days for delivery'*, but those perceptive folks in process-and-packing sixth-sensed my impatience, and within a week it arrived. I devoured the bumph on the slipcase. Bold capitals declared

'POWDER SHADERS FOR EYES. YOUR EYES ARE YOUR SOUL REFLECTORS. SOUL REFLECTORS FOR BOYS & GIRLS'

Underneath, step-by-step tutorials illustrated

'A bAsic wAy To flaTTER youR EyEs'

At the bottom, italics encouraged

> *'Be experimental because that's the only way to learn… and your man can be improved by applying a dark kohl to his inner eyelid to give that Errol Flynn look, but you might need a little help to hold him down. No doubt when he sees the results he'll be pleased with how masculine it can look.'*

Soon as I was flush, taking Toyah's advice, I skipped to Superdrug to test eyeliners. *Hmm, Miners' seem the blackest… and I'll buy a blusher an' a lipgloss…and these Funky Sprays, they look ace, especially this one.* 'Electric Azure' matched my concert trousers exactly. *I wonder if it'll be the same colour on my hair as it is on the lid?* The sales assistant's aubergine schizoid hairdo reassured me she'd have a clue. She assured me it would, and if it didn't, well it was only temporary so it would wash out easily anyway…

Home to an empty house, keen to see the bright blue me, I decided I'd do a trial run. Ready, nozzle aimed, an assertive fire… *SHIT, I MUSTA PRESSED TOO HARD!* Blue-black streamed down my brow and over my ears. My scalp looked like it was bleeding Quink, and even worse, my hair categorically *wasn't* electric azure: it was the exact same colour as the school tramp Wet Legs' pissy, washed-out navy-blue knickers. I only knew what colour Wet Legs' knickers were because she'd hike up her skirt in the middle of the playground and piss herself through her pants. The economy Sainsbury's shampoo Mom bought for me and Aidan didn't budge it, and nor did her expensive *Vidal Sassoon* one. Emergency! If Dad's nastily pungent *Head & Shoulders* was strong enough to decimate his dandruff, and it smelt strong enough to decimate the *actual* Navy, never mind some cheap navy-blue *Funky Spray*, surely that would work? But a dozen strikes of *Head & Shoulders* later, the dye still hadn't surrendered.

FUCK, POOH, BOLLOCKS! What the hell'm I gonna do?!

I had a brainwave, and doused my head in *Domestos*. Rubbing viciously, my reflected stare willing my blues away, the sand-blonde re-emerged and no wannabe New Romantic had ever felt so thrilled about looking so bland or stinking like a fresh loo. *Right, I'm gonna go an' tell that lyin' cow in the shop what's happened…*

"Shouldn'a dun that, Bab," she assessed unhelpfully. "Come to think of it tho', our Chezza's your colour an' 'er tried the blue an' it give 'er gyp too. I cor do refunds but I can swap it. Try 'Tangerine Dream', it's nearer your natural shade, if it guz wrong it won' be as noticeable."

On the big night, I'd adhered to Toyah's tips on how to attain complex eye #3 which involved gradating all four *'Soul Reflectors'* plums. I'd rimmed my inner lids, I'd been truly experimental with blusher 'til it trounced David Sylvian's, I'd lacquered my orange fringe *à la* Human League's Susanne, and every stage had gone swimmingly. My only anxiety now was *her* downstairs. She was bound to throw a wobbly, maybe even dunk me under running taps. With Rich due here in ten – an unavoidable one-off as Dad would be taxi-ing us up town – it'd be best to get it over with before he rocked up…

Mom ca-ca-cackled like an out-of-control hyaena… on-and-on…too doubled-up to form words, no *Scrub that muck off*, no *Where did you get that make-up? It better not be mine*, not even a dickybird about the smell of her *Silvikrin* which now permeated the kitchen. I rolled on more cherry lipgloss, watching her, loathing her for her reaction but equally relieved. Once she'd composed herself she sputtered, "Your hair! I've never seen anything so ridiculous in my life!"

That was out-and-out bullshit: I'd seen her '60s meringue-nest scare-styles in old snaps; then there'd been 1978's impulse Babs Streisand afro perm; and there was her current copper crop for which her hairdresser ought to be struck-off. Brought up to be honest, I reminded her again that it did her no favours…

"LESS OF YOUR LIP *CAROLINE* OR YOU SHAN'T BE GOIN' ANYWHERE!" she warned. "JOHN, COME AN' SEE *THIS!*"
Dad came in from the garden…

"'Ello sailor, give us a kiss," he propositioned, and they concertinaed in hysterics, their guffaws continuing until the doorbell rang. She beat me to it…
"You look dapper. *You're* a son any mother would be proud of," she complimented Rich on his all-black pixie boots, jeans and shirt combo. Then she subjected him to her distinct brand

of wit at my expense – performing an autopsy on my getup, declaring, "He can't be my son, not looking like that, he must be a changeling," and deciding this was the perfect moment to draw attention to my first microscopic zit *again*. To spare Rich further blushes, I piped up, "Dad, we've gotta leave *NOW!*" vowing *He's never ever coming 'round here ever again.*

At The Odeon, after traders touting costly official merchandise had bankrupted us, Rich – still as edgy as he'd been at mine – ambled towards the drabbest of the mass clogging up a lobby crackling with pre-gig anticipation.

"No, go that way, we wanna be wi' them!" I pointed at a glam squad decked out as OTT as any Newwave-NewRoPunks on *TOTP*, who were boozing more, smoking more, laughing louder and generally overdoing everything a hundredfold more than everyone else combined. They were concrete proof that thriving beneath Brum's grey overcoat was a multicolour tribe beyond that one individual – and I wasn't sure if it was a boy or a girl or some Medusa-haired Kinky-booted mutant third-sex – who'd moved into the tower block opposite Nan's. I was raring to join them, to glean beauty tips, maybe even strike up conversations and discover how they got their hair blue, pink or purple. Rich held me back by the scruff of my frilly collar…

"Nah, we ain't goin' over there, they're puffs," he scoffed. Before I could think to argue, an announcement that tonight's performance was about to start decided where we'd go.

We headed into the stalls. Rich braked at row Z.

"We won't see anythin' from here, let's push to the front," I urged, undaunted by the damage being in a sweaty throng might wreak upon my make-up.

"Nah, we don't wanna bend our programmes," he said, just as the houselights shrouded us in darkness…

Applause rippled as foggy red shafts bled through the black to reveal two guitarists and a keyboardist ad-libbing an apocalyptic intro…the drummer tossed in a familiar groove and the applause revved up fifty notches…a fierce flash shone atop an Aztec temple three storeys tall and revealed Toyah to thunderous roars…swinging from the rigging, she saluted "GOOOOOD MOOOOORNING UUUUU-NI-VER-THE" and the response blew off the Richter scale…

Haemorrhaging adrenaline, hollering

"TOY-*AAAAAAAAGGGH!*"

whatever I was experiencing as one two-thousandth of an orgiastic transaction between worshipper and worshipped equalled orgasm – minus the stress that came with four-fingers-on-thumb-street and mopping up the resultant mess.

"*C'maaan,* let's push to the front," I urged again, sure Rich *had* to be as fired up as me now Toyah had descended from her tower and hit the boards and virtually vanished from view.

"Nah, let's stay 'ere. My mom told us to be first out cuz she doesn't wanna get stuck in traffic," he said.

As every last cent I owned had been spent on a t-shirt, badge and programme, and I hadn't even the 2p bus fare home and was reliant on Mrs B's wheels, that was that. So while Toyah gave her all and I teetered on tiptoes to see her do it, he watched his Casio watch more than Toyah and continually fretted, "I hope it finishes by 10 cuz that's when my mom's comin'."

Towed away before the encore, our rock'n'roll attitudes poles apart, we sat incommunicado as Mrs B drove us home to humdrum suburbia. *'I Want to Be Free'* had never resonated truer…

Although we remained friendly at school, I didn't go 'round his 'til I called for him en route to the youth club summer disco. Clapping eyes on me in my reprised Duran state he blushed twice as feverishly as he had at mine…which was weird when Mom and Dad – who'd replayed their mickey-taking rigmarole when they'd clocked me leaving – weren't here to embarrass him. *He isn't wearing his pixie boots* I noted, striving to keep pace with him as he strode along streets ahead and answered my wittering in monosyllables. Once we were in spitting distance though, discerning

> *bop bop-bop, bop bop-bop, bop-bop,*
> *this is planet earth*

I overtook Rich, rocketed inside, and made a beeline for fellow Durannies Helen, Jo and Em, who were already throwing their best Simon Le Bon moves…

"You look fab, your hair's amazin' and – "
"your blouse is lovely and – "
"your make-up's nearly as good as Nick Rhodes's."
They rushed to complete one another's sentences, which was precisely the feedback I deserved after ninety minutes spent New Romanticizing myself. Shimmying my shoulders and jiggling my groin to *'Party Fears Two'* exactly like The Associates' sultry frontman Billy MacKenzie had done on *Razzamatazz*, I heard somebody spit "FUCKIN' QUEER" and turned my fuchsia-contoured cheek the other way; but as The Associates faded into Altered Images' *'Pinky Blue (Dance Mix)'* and I switched from being Billy to recreating singer Clare Grogan's hop-skip-jump prance, three of school's toughest Fat Knots circled, grilling

"Are they girls' clothes?"

"Why's your hair orange?"

"Does your mom know you wear make-up?"

Satisfying their curiosity as concisely as possible so I could get rid and get back to the serious business of channelling Clare, fear didn't cross my mind. They were smiling genially, after all. When they began to try and muss my hair I still wasn't afraid, gamely laughing along because, really, it *was* quite funny how I'd Silvikrin-ed it that stiff that even a wrecking ball wouldn't dent it. But seconds later, thirty fingers were getting rougher and weren't quitting even now I'd ceased laughing.

"What's the matter?" jeered one, tugging at my glittery scarf.

"We ain't gonna hurt ya," hissed number two, his homicidal stare failing to convince me a sore outcome wasn't in my stars. Now I *was* bricking it. An image flashed through my mind of them kicking three rounds of crap out of me and, if I wasn't hospitalised, of me hobbling home blue-black-and-bloody and the unsympathetic *You deserve it, looking like that* Mom would doubtless dispense once I got there. But right then, just as Fat Knot three kicked my left shin and my fears started to come true, Em, Helen and Jo, cottoned on to what was unfolding, and stepped in...

"Oi! lay off 'im!" commanded Em who had accelerated from 0 to 34CC almost overnight and become every boy's most coveted pair. Hopefully they'd obey her if it meant the teensiest possibility they'd score. The Fat Knots paused to consider. I spotted Rich watching on out of harm's way and mouthed "Help!"

"Yeah, go an' bully someone else," shooed Helen, only a cup-size behind Em, and therefore every boy's second favourite pair.

Rich strolled away...

"Yeah, leave 'im! You're just jealous cuz he's dancin' with us. And so what if he is a gay," said Jo, who, still titless, unwittingly sacrificed herself as the new target of their scorn. While the heat was off me, Jo's misfortune was my chance to bolt. With the Fat Knots on my tail howling "WE'RE GONNA BATTER YA, YA QUEER!", I tore home in an ashen sweat to prevent it becoming fact, my intestines in my mouth and my throat as arid as if it'd had antiperspirant sprayed down it, almost halving the four-minute mile.

Safely indoors, breathlessly vomiting my brush with murder as my stitches unknotted themselves, visibly and audibly shaken, the finale of what I'd foreseen did indeed play out.

"I don't blame Richard! And you deserve it, lookin' like that," said Mom.

At least now I knew whose side she was on – anybody's except mine – I'd think twice before I'd bother her with my woes again. And thank fuck school had broken up for summer because, sluggish and lonesome though the next six weeks would be without a bezzie mate, with any luck, come September – and a move to Upper School where it would be easy to lose myself – the Fat Knots would've forgotten tonight...

4

'In the church of the poison mind...'

'*Church of the Poison Mind*' Culture Club

"STANLEY, YA QUEER!"

They hadn't forgotten. Only now, to maintain the Upper School sartorial mores set by fourth and fifth year hard nuts who wore their ties thin, the Youth Club Three had already tied theirs accordingly. Quickening my speed, retying mine extra-fat, noticing that the tarts' tight skirts had gotten tighter and the tartier the hobblers the bigger the bubbles they could blow with their Hubba Bubba, dodging baby-pink balloons and ignoring "STANLEY, YA PUFF!" from older Thin Knots I hadn't even seen before, a seismic shriek stopped me in my tracks. Its architect was a Rubenesque New Romantic being attacked by a hairbrush wielded by a bull of a woman...

"WHY WON'T YOUR HAIR GO FLAT?" woofed the assailant, stoking the victim's fiery tresses ever more wildly with each heated stroke.

"I've 'ad a root perm, Miss..."
"A *WHAT?*"
"It's a special perm so I don't have to backcomb as much

to make it stay up," she translated. Such technicalities were plainly foreign to the grey-cropped frump.

"YOU KNOW IT IS STRICTLY FORBIDDEN FOR GIRLS TO PERM OR COLOUR THEIR HAIR!" raged The Bull. This smacked of victimisation when, all around us, I could count more burgundy rinses and poodle perms than Mom'd given us whacks. "WASH IT OUT TONIGHT OR YOU'LL BE IN BIG TROUBLE!"

"I can't, Miss, it's permanent."

"IN THAT CASE YOU'VE EARNED YOURSELF A WEEK'S DETENTION! AND SCRUB THAT MUCK OFF YOUR FACE, YOU LOOK LIKE A CLOWN!"

I'd heard that before. I bet when Mom had taught at Seniors she'd said exactly the same thing. Imagining the bane to beauty Mrs Stanley must've been, how if girls had dared answer back "But you've got tons of make-up on and *your* hair's dyed, Miss" she would've bawled "DO AS I SAY, NOT AS I DO!" because that's what she'd always yell at me, I knew that – as unjust as *my* school's bane to glamour was – at least she wasn't a hypocrite.

The Bull charged at some other luckless lass whose law-breaking hoop earrings had suddenly beckoned like a red rag. The shrieker was giving the finger to a gaggle of gum-poppers who'd been sniggering over Miss's shoulder throughout her inhumane ordeal. I was anxious to talk to her, and although this probably wasn't the ideal time to approach her, especially since she'd just sworn at some cretin who'd called her a weirdo, I'd waited too fucking long to befriend a New Romantic. Steeled for the worst I strode boldly over, leaping straight in with a hair compliment to break the ice. The flame-maned heavyweight stared stonily, as if waiting for some sarky P.S. that would entitle her to deck an oick half her size…

"And your make-up's the best I've ever seen," I said to butter her up. That wasn't me being desperately sycophantic, because hers sincerely was: spotlessly applied opaque pancake foundation, tiny eyes skilfully maximized in metallic shadows winged across her temples to her hairline, absent cheekbones deftly forged in bronze. That did it. Her angular lip-liner softened to a smile and, with her defences dropped, she was almost as stunning as Kate Haysi Fantayzee.

"Thanks. If that dyke expects me to wash it off she can kiss my arse. An' I'm gonna backcomb my bloody hair every bloody day just to piss her off...thank God I'll be outta this bloody dump in a few months...soz, I'm Ronnie. What's your name?"

As the bell rudely interrupted her, she added, "Meet us here at break...if you wanna risk gettin' in trouble for talkin' to me!"

Ronnie was with her brawny pal Sandra. She was nowhere near as gorge as Ronnie – partly due to a hostile sneer that gave the impression she had a harelip. Her make-up wasn't as perfect either – mainly down to dense bum-fluff that prevented her pan-stick sitting smooth. Nonetheless, her Flock of Seagulls' wedge-cut and whiplash eyeliner were sufficiently New Romantic to enthrall me. The exotic duo divulged insider info on where they and their ilk did their clothes shopping: a chic backstreet boutique called Kahn & Bell; The Rag Market's second-hand stalls; Oasis, a four-floor megastore which catered mainly to Goths and sounded right up my street now that I was into Siouxsie and the Banshees with a vengeance. I'd even white-lied to Mom that my new school shoes cost more than they did, then 'lost' the receipt and spent the rest on a Siouxsie best-of. They regaled me with tales about *The Holy City Zoo* – an achingly hip nightspot they frequented where a top night out was out-posing the competition to a playlist of Bowie, Roxy, Disco and NewRo, and where boys wore more make-up than girls and boys snogged boys and girls kissed girls and drunk Sandra had even slipped Ronnie the tongue once – and the veteran clubbers had only just moved on to telling me about Barbarellas, where they'd seen an unknown DuranDuran play, when an irate

"STANLEY, HERE! NOW!"

snatched me back to mundanity. It was our perma-tanned silver fox headmaster, Mr McLaughlin...

"What are *those* things on your feet?"
I glanced at my point-toe side-lace winkle pickers.
"Erm... shoes, sir."
"Don't be obnoxious! They are NOT appropriate footwear! I do NOT want to see you wearing them again."

Before I could enquire if pixie boots would be okay, he tore away in pursuit of a skinhead with a super-skinny knot and calf-high cherry DMs. I guessed it'd be wisest to keep me and my winkle pickers out of McLaughlin's way, and flee in the opposite direction or duck behind Ronnie whenever he was in the vicinity, to try and stay low-key. And if Boy George hadn't happened I might've succeeded...

I'd never regarded myself remotely pretty until, filling a Sunday comparing my reflection to Boy George's pic on the cover of *'Kissing To Be Clever'*, I'd detected a definite resemblance. The press had dubbed him 'gender bender', and the Thin Knots had seized it and would shout it each time they saw me, and although it made staying low-key increasingly difficult, I took it for the flattery they didn't intend. A boy had to find flattery wherever he could. Particularly when Mom continued to make me feel shit by zooming-in on my sporadic zits like I hadn't already spotted them, and vainly tried to squeeze them gone so she wouldn't have anything to pick on. The more I harassed them the angrier they grew, which left me feeling even shittier. Marilyn Monroe could stick her diamonds; *Miners* cover-stick was this boy's best friend.

I wasn't so ecstatic when the Thin Knots curtailed 'gender bender' to "BENDER!" though, even less so once that swelled into the emphatically unflattering "STANLEY, YA FUCKIN' BENDER!" But I was resolute I wouldn't show them they were getting to me. And I didn't 'til the April day they accidentally-on-purpose bumped me in the corridor and I took a tumble and my bag spewed books much to their amusement and I lost my cool and flipped

"FUCK OFF, YOU IDIOTS!"

"STANLEY!"

The Thin Knots scarpered. As I scooped up my stuff, McLaughlin, standing over me, barked, "I will *NOT* tolerate profanity in my school!"

"But they swore at me first!"

"Quiet! I didn't give you permission to speak. It's you I heard swearing!"

"But they've been bullying – "

"Shut up! My wife and I saw you in Solihull last Saturday dressed like a girl and we were appalled. Your parents might not care how you dress or what language you use but – "

"But I only swore at them because – "

"Don't interrupt! If you are being bullied, and it's highly unlikely – "

"BUT I AM!"

47

"DO *NOT* RAISE YOUR VOICE TO ME! AND DON'T INTERRUPT! You swear, you are disrespectful, I told you those shoes contravene uniform rules yet you're *still* wearing them… report to me for detention at home-time!"

Put in the pokey First Aid room, resenting McLaughlin for disciplining me because I didn't comply with his criteria of how boys should be, straying from the exercise he'd set me, I furiously stabbed down a few adjectives that fit him:

> Loathsome
> Objectionable
> Unfair
> Creep
> Hideous

Chewing my pen lid, humming *'Church Of The Poison Mind'*, my thoughts roamed. *If this hellhole were a church school it'd be the church of poisoned minds, not C of E, 'cause all the teachers an' pupils are free to preach the gospel according to McLaughlin on the likes of Ronnie an' me…*
I'd abstractedly overwritten the first letter of each considered word. A sixth word leapt out: LOUCH. Saying it out loud, its spiteful sound summed him up in one. In this church, 'LOUCH' was an apt moniker for its head.

Mom didn't ask why I was late when I got home. Loath though I was to fill her in when I was 99.9 per cent positive what she'd say, seeing as there was still that 0.1 per cent possibility she'd be sympathetic, I relayed the whole story, from being bollocked for my winkle-pickers right through to being unfairly punished when *I'd* been the one being bullied.
"I said those aren't suitable school shoes but you have to be different, don't you? No wonder they tease you! God,

it's like when you came home crying after your first day at Infants' – I told you they'd laugh at you going in your cowboy outfit but you wouldn't listen, would you?! And knowing what a mouthy Smart Alec you are, you deserved detention. It's a good job you've got that theatre trip tomorrow, you won't be able to rile...and his name's Mr McLaughlin, not Louch!"

So that was that. There *really* wouldn't be any point bothering her with my problems again.

Boarding the coach next morning, I honoured a hushed "Bender" – from Alan of all people – with a similarly hushed "It takes one to know one," then joined the girls at the back, resolving I'd react as serenely to any other slurs that day. But once we hit the motorway and the calls of *Stanley you fucking bender* got underway, I answered the ninth slur with a full-throttle, "FUCK YOU, YOU STUPID TWAT!"

"MR STANLEY!" boomed Mrs Corner, aka Rent-a-Tent, lumbering up the gangway as fast as her chafing thighs could carry her. "FRONT, NOW!"
"S'not fair, they started it..."

"I DON'T CARE. MOVE YOURSELF!"

No sooner did Rent-a-Tent install me across from her and wedge her four-berth bulk back into a seat meant for two, than she had to heave herself out to investigate another rumpus. I'd already noticed my neighbour's bottle-black *Dennis the Menace* hairstyle and the Siouxsie badge pinned to her ample bosom, and with Rent-a-Tent gone I introduced myself.

"A'right Carl, you troublemaker, I'm Kayleigh."

"I love your hair! What's up with your face though? It looks like it's been Black'n'Deckered!"

"Thanks a bunch… I think I'm becomin' allergic to school soap…Mottram's a right cow makin' me take my make-up off, I did it really good today too, proper Siouxsie…d'ya like Siouxsie?"

Exhibit one: I showed her my Siouxsie badge.

Then the circumstantial evidence: "My uncle was into Siouxsie. He died, my Nan gave me his records and there were some Banshees' singles amongst them…I only got into them properly recently though…bought their old albums…and a Siouxsie t-shirt from that shop Oasis…d'you know Oasis?"

She nodded.

"I got some bondage trousers from Oasis too," I bragged, returning the dialogue to Kayleigh by questioning why I'd never seen her around.

"Cuz I skive a lot. An' when I *am* there, I keep myself to myself cuz everybody hates me an' I hate them," she explained impassively.

My line of vision had travelled up her face and was rested covetously on her Goth crowning glory. Reading my mind, she generously volunteered, "I'll dye yours if ya wanna. Come 'round to ours on Saturday."

Rent-a-Tent came thudding back, puffing some sarcasm at Kayleigh that as she'd been ticked off once today for turning up in Halloween fancy dress, if she had an ounce of common-sense and didn't want to be deposited on the hard shoulder, she'd do well to remember we were going to Coventry and send eloquent Mr Stanley to Coventry and not engage in his conversation. That was fine though, because we'd said all we needed for now. As I watched the arduous farce being hammed up onstage, I mulled over Kayleigh's proposal. I'd been shilly-shallying about crossing to *the dark side* for weeks, worried it mightn't suit me when Mom liked to remind me – and often – that I'd been born an 'ugly black-haired rat'. Though it was in glorious Technicolor, the lone photo there was in existence of her hesitantly cradling the week-old me was too blurry to make out whether black hair would suit me or not, but by curtain call, my decision was made all the same...

Twitchy as a child on a long excursion mithering *Are we there yet?* I tested Kayleigh's patience every-minute-on-the-minute by pestering "Is it ready yet?" Finally – after thirty progressively testy No's – it was. Kayleigh rinsed it and towel-dried it, then for maximum impact she turban-tied the towel and guided me to the mirrored medicine cabinet. With a fanfare of "*Tah-dah!*" she whipped the towel away.

"O-H......M-Y......G-O-D!!!!!"
"Don't say you hate it cuz it's a bit late if you do."
"NO! I *adore* it!"

She led me back to her room, slathered my hair in a supersize dollop of sheer-green Boots *Country Style Setting Gel*, blow-dried it into spikes, and cemented them with Boots' own-brand extra-firm hairspray with the pink lid, recommending I get a can as it was top of the market. She wasn't done yet though, not when what became Goths most weren't anaemic brows and lashes. Sharpening her tool, psycho-kohler Kayleigh went on a heavy-handed rampage, going in for the kill with liquid liner 'til she'd snuffed out every blonde trace, then handing me a hand-mirror to inspect the damage.
"Whaddya reckon?" she fished.

Spellbound by this familiar foreigner, absorbing his slug eyebrows and Egyptian eyes, "I... I... I... I..." I couldn't express my joy I was that elated – elated because I'd always resembled Mom, yet now we didn't even look related! God knows what she'd say. Reluctant as I was to subject Kayleigh to Mom's scathing tongue, I trusted that her appearance would render Mom blind to me.

"Hey," I suggested, "shall we go to mine?"

I let Kayleigh go in first, directing her to the kitchen where Mom was hunched over her newspaper. "Who are you?" demanded Mom; but before Kayleigh could reply, Mom spied me hovering in the hall, and howled so hysterically she slid off her chair. Composure regained, in one breath she managed to re-air the 'ugly black-haired rat' anecdote *and* compliment Kayleigh's Goth façade *and* decry mine *and* ask, "Why the hell would you want to do that to yourself?"

But her question must've been rhetorical; because without waiting for an explanation I didn't have she'd already turned away from home affairs and returned to more crucial current affairs, like Maggie's re-election victory. As I passed Dad on the driveway – with not the slightest flicker from him to suggest he'd even registered my makeover – he cheerily enquired, "Will you be in for dinner?"

"He ain't very observant is he?" observed Kayleigh archly. "Can't believe he didn't say anythin'. Even *my* dad noticed when I started dressin' different!"

"Yeah, everyone'll have lots to say at school though," I laughed.

They didn't have long to say it though. Almost the second I set foot inside, livid Louch had frogmarched me out and across the playground – and as he thrust me off the premises he gunned "I DON'T WANT TO SEE YOU HERE AGAIN UNTIL YOU ARE NORMAL!"

That'll mean either stayin' at home 'til it grows out or shaving it off…an' I know what Mom'll make me do. For a while I roamed the streets in a panic about the humiliation of walking into school bald tomorrow, but a feeling of *carpe diem* soon prevailed. I took the bus into town. I only had 53½p, but I was blessed with a capacious bag and the gall to fill it, so I went to the flagship Boots to shoplift what I couldn't afford – my trusty *Miners* concealer and eye pencil, a *Leichner Kamera Klear* foundation in palest ivory, a translucent *Max Factor Crème Puff*, a *Mary Quant* black lippy, a *No 7* liquid liner like Kayleigh had used and her preferred hairspray – prior to descending into the nearby Gents to get ready for Oasis…

I zhuzhed my hair and deadened my face, and – struggling to master that slippery fluid eyeliner – I fucked my left eye up when a geriatric perv with the charisma of Frank Carson unexpectedly surfaced from a lock-up cock-in-hand and solicited, "Wanna suck this, Sonny Jim?" Repulsed to think that *anyone* would do that in a pissy public loo, let alone mistake me for the sort of boy who would, I sent him packing with a blasphemous negative, conceding *I'd have said yes if it was Matthew Ashman asking.* I de-schooled that tell-tale uniform by threading my tie through my belt loops and turning my blazer inside out. And I was navigating Oasis's labyrinthine fly-posted stairwells and walkways, lost in my own little world, thinking how fucking superb I looked, when the harmonious patchouli-heavy ambiance which always pervaded this haven for the dispossessed was invaded by an *Adidas* eyesore blazing around a corner, threatening, "Fuckin' touch me an' you're fuckin' dead you fuckin' freak!"

Hot on his heels speed-limped a one-shoed lanky she-male sheathed in a silver-blue body-stocking – her-his scalp entirely shaved save for a waist-length platinum ponytail flowing from a skinny tube rising from her-his crown a perfectly perpendicular foot; acute angle brows crooking a 'V' at Mother Nature; and a hundredweight of hoops hanging from her-his ears and nostrils. Flailing her-his other skyscraper stiletto scythe-like, her-his sole objective evidently GBH, this extra-terrestrial Boudicca was spurred along by stallholders – Goths, Punks, Psychobillies and Cyberfreaks shaking their fists, baying "GET HIM! GET HIM!"

Very shortly she/he re-emerged unruffled, checking her-his shoe wasn't damaged, broadcasting in unquestionably male bass Brummie, "Thar'll teach 'im not t' cum in 'ere takin' the piss ourra me." The wail of an ambulance arriving outside proved *Hell hath no fury like a tranny scorned* and was celebrated with high fives from his co-workers for having single-footedly seen-off his tormentor. Eager to speak to him, I stalked him to the basement eatery, a grotty establishment with grubby Formica tables where – as I'd learnt the hard way when a hot dog had left me nauseous after my first visit – the grub spoke for itself ad nauseam and none but the Teflon-stomached ate twice.

I'd found it challenging enough to get my hair to stick up at all, so I was flummoxed by how he'd managed to attach that towering pole to his pate and engineered it so it would defy physics, and I studied him as he sugared his takeaway tea at the counter. I couldn't quite place the *hows* or *wheres*, but I definitely recognised him from somewhere. It wasn't Oasis though, because I'd never seen him here. Catching me gawking, as he sashayed out he crossed his eyes and gurned, which didn't deter me from following…

The object of my investigation stalled at the stall special-ising in leather and PVC, everything from simple vests to harnesses which – without bodies to make sense of them – were baffling on-the-hanger. As I fingered a three-tier studded belt, he saw the opportunity for a sale, and asked

"Yow awlroight there, doyer?"

"Yeah, just lookin'. I'm broke. Hey, I'm sure I know you but…"

"Evereewon duz, doyer, oi've bin arowund fer yeaers. Yow'll 'uv sin me in the noight clubs."

"Nah, I haven't been to a club yet."

"Maybe yow've sin me arowund Smethwick then, oi've gorra flat there with me 'usband Bri."

The penny dropped.

"Not Windmill Lane?"

It transpired he was that fantastical creature who lived on the estate where Nan had lived before she'd been re-housed three years ago, and Ray knew who Nan was because she service-washed his and Bri's smalls.

"Oh God, if you see her don't tell her you saw us, she might tell my mom an' I'm supposed to be in school, but my headmaster chucked me out 'cause of my hair and –"

"Dow worry, doyer, oi woe say a word," he promised, and he winked conspiratorially as he slipped the belt into my bag with a covert, "An' doe yow goo tellin' anyone oi gave you this!"

Next morning, a pillow, a duvet and a shut bedroom door couldn't stymie Mom's dulcet tones. Every couple of minutes she playfully crowed "Rise an' shine, wakey-wakey sunshine!"

– she'd had a good seeing-to last night – until eventually she burst in and angrily drew back the curtains, shouting,

"SHIFT YOURSELF YOU LAZY IGNORAMUS OR YOU'LL BE LATE!"

"I'm not going," I yawned, cursing the sun and burrowing under the bedclothes.

"RUBBISH, YOU'RE NOT ILL," she pooh-poohed, like that would've made an iota of difference.

Aged six, I'd punched a windowpane, certain that cuts would spell time away from Abi's teasing; this year I'd emptied a boiling kettle on my foot hoping third-degree burns would warrant a break from the Thin Knots; both self-inflictions had resulted in me being driven to school direct from A&E; and I'd learned that nothing but decapitation was likely to earn me a sick day.

Mom instigated a duvet tug-o'-war I was determined to win to hide this morning's fresh sticky patch and last week's crusty dozen. In a weak position and close to losing, I had only one shot to disarm her: I blurted what Louch had done yesterday. She let go.

"HE DID *WHAT*? RIGHT! UP, NOW! I WANT YOU IN THE CAR IN ONE MINUTE!"

When she raced three amber lights and swerved a right towards school rather than straight ahead to the barbers I sensed something strange was afoot. She braked just short of ploughing into the pebbledash, and, as I raced to keep up, we gate-crashed Louch's office before his secretary could stop us...

"C-c-can I-I-I h-h-help y-y-you?" stuttered Louch, cowering in his chair behind his desk.

56

Spike heels impaled in the rug, her nails ingrained in the wood, immovable Mom leant across and flared, "ARE YOU GOING TO THROW ME OUT FOR HAVING DYED HAIR TOO, *MR MCLAUGHLIN?*"

Catatonic, Louch looked to me. I shrugged. I was as shocked as him.

"Well, what's the matter? Has the cat got your tongue? I'm telling you now – black hair or no black hair – he's staying. Because if you think you can remove one of your top pupils just for dyeing his hair then I'll be taking this all the way to the board of governors," she carried on, defending her terminally-dyed son's right-to-dye.

"And *don't* try soft soaping me! Twelve years I've worked in education! I know the correct procedure for expelling pupils an' it's not done without going through the appropriate channels. Right, I think we understand each other, don't we? That's all I've come to say. Have a nice day, *S-I-I-R*," she bade derisively, spinning on a ha'penny and swanning out…

"Does that mean I've gotta stay?" I checked, uncertain if the wills of headmasters could be overruled and hopeful that they couldn't.

"Get to class," glared Louch.

Being forced to stay was the worst punishment I could have had. There was only one real loser in this battle: me.

5

'A wild celebration of feelings inside...'

'Soul Inside' Soft Cell

Mom had fetched the authentic artificial spruce from the loft a fortnight ago. It had stood naked in the front living-room a good week before she'd said, "C'mon sunshine, you love decorating it, let's do it together, get ourselves in the festive spirit." *Oh, she's talkin' to me again* I'd thought...

For weeks she'd been giving me the silent treatment for a) dying the bathroom carpet black – in actuality an imperceptible speck, and b) for returning home with a cobweb-knit black sweater after she'd made me pledge I'd spend the child allowance she'd entrusted me with on something sensible for winter. When I'd shown it to her she'd erupted, yelling that it would be impractical in sub-zero temperatures. As if boring practicalities like warmth mattered.

"It's *my* child allowance, I can spend it on what I want," I'd argued.

"NO, IT'S MY CHILD ALLOWANCE, IT'S PAID TO ME. I CARRIED YOU FOR NINE MONTHS," she'd retaliated.

In previous years I wouldn't have had to be asked to decorate the tree but – since I'd become a Goth – baubles, tinsel and fairy-lights just weren't me anymore. She'd have been wasting her breath asking Aidan or Dad to help out, so in the end she'd done it herself, along with Sellotaping the hundred-odd cards sent to 'Janet, John, Aidan and Carl' to lengths of silver thread and hanging them. She'd moaned about it of course, but like I'd told her, "I didn't ask for a bloody tree an' they're not my bloody cards!" No, my only concession to Christmas thus far had been shoplifting gifts; and my only other concession would be to greedily unwrap my presents and play Siouxsie and the Banshees' *'Il est Né Le Divin Enfant'*, a Gallic carol with bells and muted horns which revealed their softer side. Should she start on me again though, I'd blast that cacophonous Banshees' rant that beseeched *'Fuck the mothers kill the others, kill the mothers fuck the others'* instead...

Kayleigh had started dating this guy, Seb. We'd met briefly outside the school gates when he'd come to meet her. He was nineteen, with ebony spiked hair, razor-sharp cheek-bones and inviting lips, shrink-wrapped in the skinniest drainpipes that required zilch effort to see which side he dressed and a hip-slung belt buckle resting provocatively on his bulge. I'd automatically fallen in lust and hadn't stopped wanking over him since.

The first Saturday of the holidays, Kayleigh rang to tell me they'd collect me in an hour. I put on my gloomiest Goth glad-rags – black peg-top trousers, a batwing top I'd run-up on Mom's antique black-and-gold Singer sewing machine she'd inherited from her gran, and that cobweb jumper – and took extra care over my make-up to make an impact on Seb. When I saw his decidedly un-Goth daffodil Capri swerve onto our drive my heart cartwheeled like we were going on a date...

Seb, the perfect gentleman, got out to let me in – placing a cheeky hand on my bum and stealing an ungentlemanly squeeze as I clambered into the backseat. Before we set off, he offered me a fag. I didn't smoke, hadn't ever even tried, but I took one anyway. He held up his lit lighter and, unused to the mechanics of sparking up, I blew...

"You've gotta suck," he smirked, staring me out as he reignited the flame. *Mmmmm, I'd love to,* I fantasized, drawing too hard and coughing up my guts...

"Not that 'ard," mocked Kayleigh, reminding me she was here too. I positioned myself behind the driver's seat so I could see Seb's sexy hazel eyes in the rear-view mirror, his focus flitting between me and the road. With carbon monoxide filling my lungs and sex filling my mind it was definitely goodbye to Sandra Dee...

First on our itinerary was a tour of Oasis. Seb stopped to chat to an acquaintance who'd patched-up her hangover to haul herself here at the crack of noon to promote The Zig Zag – *the* happeningest club nowanights apparently, to where she gave him three 'FREE B4 10' fliers – and I exchanged smalltalk with Ray.

"*You* know Beanpole Ray? Ray's, like, the Queen Mother of the scene," said Kayleigh.

"Yeah, we've been friends for years," I lied.

And up went my cred.

Seb advocated we head to Rackhams, town's swankiest department store. Apparently, its sixth floor café was where the Alternative in-crowd went to see-and-be-seen every Saturday.

"They can be brutal if you're a first-timer," he forewarned. "They won't tell you if they think you look good but if they think you look crap they'll chase you straight out."

The merciless jurors – over forty of them – preened to perfection and taking up a quarter of the seats, scrutinised me silently, their blank faces betraying nada. As soon as they resumed their banter I could relax. I'd passed. Unlike the sloppy Gothette whose patchily-dyed skew-whiff Mohican, errant eyeliner and generally rotten demeanour raised an onslaught of *woofs*...

"This isn't a zoo, I've paid to dine here in peace!" trumpeted a twinset-and-pearls patron, only for a gobby Mohawk to snap, "If you don't like it here, bog off you fat snobby cow."

"Why, I have never been so insulted – "

"With that minging face I'm sure you have, luv," butted in another. Twinset clicked her fingers at a tray collector and demanded, "Fetch your manager!"

He arrived, ignored the fact that our entire freak-show was sharing just five beverages between them, and unsympathetically directed her elsewhere. "There are two other cafés on floors one and two, madam," he told her, as a pack of Punks hounded the unfortunate Gothette out, yapping "FUCKIN' DOG!"

Twinset, who should've felt privileged she could witness this selection process which upheld the underground scene's lofty standards, and all for the cost of a finger roll and a *Douwe Egbert* filter coffee, waddled away foaming, "You heathens need National Service!"

"Did you see the state of that girl...she deserves it...at least if they've made her cry she won't ruin her make-up," I bitched.

"You've fit right in, 'aven't you? I hope I ain't created a monster cuz you was so sweet 'til I got my hands on you and Seb brung you here!"

Mooning over Seb, sourly thinking *What's Kayleigh got that I haven't? I'm prettier, I'm funnier AND I'm thin* over two more cups of tea, when she mooted we go somewhere else for a drink, I groaned, "But we've had three."

"No, I mean alcohol, ya knobhead!"

So we trudged to some rock'n'roll dive, went directly to the Ladies to refresh our hair and make-up, and were interrupted by a tattooed pit-bull of a bloke who bulldozed in snarling "OUT! I DON'T WANT ANY FUCKIN' PUFFS IN MY PUB!"

"Fuck him. There's this place 'round the corner, I prefer it there anyway," said Seb.

Its discreet entrance was nestled between a Balti house and a cinema. Seb pressed a buzzer marked *'Legends'* and a woman instructed "Pull hard, Bab." We climbed winding stairs, and Seb buzzed a second intercom. Fort Knox would've been easier to break into, but we were in at last...

The place was festooned for the festive season like Liberace had been let loose. Beneath the spangles and illuminations that outshone Blackpool's were silvery flocked walls hung with framed black-and-whites of Streisand, Garland, and every other camp icon. Broadway tunes blared. Four manly women were supping pints. A cackle of womanly men were camping it up to Ethel Merman. A moustachioed barman was dressed like a Village Person in a tinsel-trimmed leather cap, sleeveless plaid shirt and tight snow-washed jeans hoicked so high to flaunt his crown jewels that they made *my* balls hurt. An Ethel Merman whooped, "When you've served these lovely folks, I'll have two G 'n' T's with ice 'n' a slice, a Legover and half a lager 'n' lime please, Mother!"

Seb had brought us to a gay bar. The denim-clad blokey bloke at the bar who'd have fit in better at a Status Quo convention was the single un-gay thing in here…

"What can I do you for, Bab?" tooted Mother, lips tighter than a cat's sphincter, who – as he was manning the show alone – I deduced must be the woman who'd buzzed us in.

"Whaddya fancy, Stan?" asked Seb, stroking my arse.

Stan? No one's called me 'Stan' before…if Seb likes it tho' that's what I'll call myself from now on I decided, scanning the bewildering array of beers and optics. Seeing too many options, and not wanting to choose the wrong one, I said, "I'll have whatever you're having."

As Mother prepared three double-vodka oranges, Seb suddenly straightened up, took his roving fingers off me, and full-on snogged Kayleigh. Glasses dry, Seb ordered another round and Kayleigh and I sat down…

"That guy in the denim must fancy you cuz he keeps starin'," reckoned Kayleigh.

"Eugh, I hope not! He's ancient, he's gotta be thirty, *and* he's ginger," I sneered, disowning my natural hue. "I don't fancy him at all, or anyone else here…" *Except Seb.*

When Kayleigh told Seb "Stan's got an admirer," he told me to ignore Mr Denim and killed that topic by saying we should go to The Zig Zag later. Would I get in, I questioned. Yes, guaranteed Seb. And as it didn't close 'til 2, I should 'phone my mom at some point to tell her that I'd be late home, Kayleigh added. No need I replied: we weren't talking, she didn't give a shit about me and she'd be glad I wasn't there.

That was sorted then, we'd stay here until The Zig Zag opened at 9. Kayleigh and Seb started snogging again. Looking here-there-and-anywhere to avoid looking at them, noticing Mr Denim was still staring, I decided that –

fancy him or not – the least his tenacity deserved was a slight
smile. That was all the encouragement he needed to stagger
over...

"Was yooer neyem? How auld aar ya? Y'bin heeuh
befawa?" he slurred; but without waiting for answers,
he tapped my empty and asked, "Was at yas drink'n?"

I wasn't about to pass up a freebie just because he didn't
float my boat. He stumbled to the bar, stumbled back,
and since Seb and Kayleigh were still snogging and I'm a
chatterbox and he was somebody to chat to, I drained my glass
in one and belatedly answered, "I'm Stan, I'm fourteen,
and I'm a *Legends* virgin."

Something I'd said seemed to excite him. He lunged at
me, more in control of his tongue than his legs, my taste
buds wincing at the sharp sweet tang of his neat whisky. My
knee-jerk reaction was to fight him off, but, granting that he
had bought me a double-vodka and there probably was no
such thing as a free drink in a gay bar, it seemed only right to
oblige. Surprised by how gently he kissed for a gruff Geordie
with stubble and 'HATE' tattooed on both sets of knuckles, I
was just getting into my first male kiss when he drew away to
ask, "Aar yas butch er bitch?"

"Well, I can be a bit of a bitch sometimes," I said.

Kayleigh and Seb pissed themselves laughing. Mr Denim,
puzzled, hauled himself off the sofa and swayed to the bar.

"What's so funny? I don't get it, tell me!" I implored,
squiffy from three large vodkas. They didn't explain, and
returned to eating face instead. Soon, Mr Denim had slumped
beside me with a fourth double. Knocking it straight back,
finding him increasingly attractive through vodka glasses,

now *I* pounced on *him*…frantic kisses…my inquisitive mitts moving to investigate his crotch. It was massive. And my fervent fingers might have unleashed the beast within had Seb not interrupted me, "Stan! The Zig Zag's open, we're off."

"Okay, I'm coming," I obeyed.

Mr Denim gripped my wrist tight and growled intimidatingly, "Yad bettor cum back, aaal the brass aah've spent on yoo. Coss if yoo dooun't an' aah ivver see yoo agyen al fucken' kill yoo."

The psycho believed it when I lied I would. He loosened his hold, and I ran after Seb and Kayleigh…

At the bottom of the stairs, Kayleigh advised, "Fix your lippy cuz it's smudged…unless you wanna look like Robert Smith!" I didn't. As I rummaged in my bag for my lipstick, thinking *I'm really lucky having a friend like Kayleigh or I'd have walked into the club looking crap*, Seb reprimanded, "That bloke could've been a queer-basher. Don't kiss anyone else tonight, alright?"

"Okay," I promised, thinking *And I'm really lucky Seb's looking out for me too…God, I'm hammered, hope we haven't gotta walk far…*

Thankfully it was only ten doors down. Stepping into the uncharted nightlife I'd waited a year to experience ever since Ronnie had first told me about it, this spartan red-lit cavity with its dancer-less dancefloor, gummy carpet, filthy furniture and four punters propping up a bar running the length of the far wall was an extreme anti-climax.

"Is this it?" I pouted.

"Don't worry, it'll be busy in a bit," promised Seb.

Two double vodkas later, it was jammed with expected Punks etcetera and unexpected dreadlock Rastas lolling around smoking funny-smelling roll-ups. Beanpole Ray arrived wearing a leather micro-mini, a bustier, fishnets, sky-high gladiator boots, straps up his arms, a gigantic lion's-head-clasp belt and several more of those unfathomably attached tubes. Tonight he had black and orange ponytails sprouting from his head. Seb presented me to some nameless dandy, whispering, "His cock's enormous, it's got a gorgeous shiny red end." He didn't clarify how he knew though. Then he introduced me to Gay John who – with his floppy Brylcreem-ed quiff and a bare six-pack that oozed sex – was the dishiest man I'd ever set eyes on. Gay John was with Whiskers – a rugged Rockabilly with the bushiest sideburns imaginable – who looked as straight as they come but wasn't because he had an equally rugged boyfriend. They were with Mad Sarah, barking at the moon and glued to her unrequited love Patti Bell, half of the *Kahn & Bell* Ronnie had told me about, whose rainbow hair-extensions must've weighed half her bodyweight.

"She's gotta be forty but look at her face an' figure," murmured Kayleigh deferentially.

"No way, she could be eighteen! She must have a picture in her attic, I bet her real name's Doreen Gray," I joked.

And over there was Twiggy – sporting the same unfathomably attached tubes as Beanpole Ray, and dressed and made-up identically. Only Twiggy was shorter, prettier and even thinner. Seb said they'd been bickering forever as to who had invented the look first, although as Brum's Alternative scene had practically come into being purely to give Ray somewhere to go he *had* to claim credit. I was glad I'd been versed in club politics. It might be tricky being pally with both.

Kayleigh and I went to dance, slaving to keep up with the DJ's offbeat set that oscillated from The Cramps' schlock-horror Pyschobilly-skiffle to New Order; from vintage punk to Grace Jones' lithe reggae-funk; from Arthur Brown's *'Fire'* to high-energy disco – the gargantuan drag-diva Divine's demand to *'Dance, rock, feel the beat, rock your body to the native beat'* inciting a sudden stampede onto an already saturated dancefloor fogged in dry ice. My make-up melting and a bladderful of booze, Kayleigh pointed me to the Ladies, which was "More fun than the Gents" apparently.

Since when are toilets meant to be 'fun'? I wondered as I pushed my way in…

Exquisite girls and boys, and – under unforgiving fluorescent strips – a fair few munters, were all vying for precious mirror space through a hazardous hairspray haze that miraculously didn't ignite from all the fags being lit. Embellishing who'd done what to whom or elucidating who they wanted to do as they retouched their make-up, they were being jostled by those who'd come or had been to answer the call of nature, shoving in-and-out of cubicles, some of them in groups. *Why does it take so many people to piss? And why's it taking them so bloody long? Wish they'd hurry up, I'm touching cloth!* A door swung open and a fingerless lace-gloved hand pulled me in…

Its flamboyant owner – an ageless blonde reincarnation of Valeria from *Carry on Screaming* – drawled, "Sliiide the lock, deeear…be a daaarling and hold this!"

She handed me her purse, fiddling in her handbag and jabbering, "Bear with me daaarling…I won't be a mo… I caaan't have dropped it, thaaat would be an absoloootely terrible waste of fifty pounds!"

I could buy twenty-five twelve inches for that! What's she lost – a diamond ring? Fuck, if I don't piss soon I'll…

"Er, I really need to…d'you mind if I…"

"Nooooo, be my guest!"

I handed her back her purse and manoeuvred around her to wee. I'd scarcely finished pissing when she squealed, "I'VE FOUND IT!" and manoeuvred around me to wipe the cistern lid with loo roll. I'd no idea what would come next, and I observed her as she carefully unwrapped "my weekly prezzie to myself" and softly tapped an album's-worth of the pricey powder onto the cistern and separated it into two lines with a bank card. She handed me a miniature silver straw.

"What's *this* for?"

"You've n-e-v-e-r done cocaine?! How quaint! Daaarling, watch me!"

Pressing her left nostril with her left index finger, she sniffed with her right nostril, sniffed again as she rose, and passed me the straw…

I did what she'd done. Nothing seemed to change.

"How's that, daaarling?"

"I don't feel any different…"

"Oh, you will!"

As she put her paraphernalia in order, I complimented her plunge-neck ruched skin-tight white number.

"Thank you, daaarling. I treated myself for Christmas. It's a Patti Bell. Patti's *sooo* talented and she's *sooo* beautiful and *sooo* diviiine…do you know Patti?"

"Yeah, of course I do," I embroidered – omitting to mention 'know' meant I knew who she was.

"In that case, let's have another line, daaarling…a nice *BIIIG* one…thisss will keep you awake *all* night!"

After we'd hoovered up that, she rewrapped the cocaine, tucked it safely in her purse, *mwah-mwah'd* "Merry Christmas" and out we slipped. Seb, first-in-line for the loo, pushed me back in, bolted the door, slammed me against the wall and thrust his tongue in, circling it slowly and passionately, his lips heavenly soft. Gratefully capitulating for the longest time but becoming unusually dominant once I'd surreptitiously swallowed the bitter mucus that had slid from my sinuses, now I slammed him against the opposite wall...voraciously exploring his mouth's every crevice...harder and deeper... massaging his hard-on through his trousers...Seb somehow asking, while his mouth was otherwise engaged, "Are you in love with me?"

"Whatever 'in love' means," I cockily retorted, Prince Charles style.

"What does that mean? You either are or you aren't."

"Of course I am! I love you!"

Grinning, he suddenly straightened up like he'd done at *Legends*, and said, "I should find Kayleigh."

Remembering Kayleigh's advice *vis-à-vis* smudged lipstick, I wiped mine off her boyfriend, vacated the lock-up, stopped at the mirrors to reapply, then went back to the dancefloor... my throat numb, heartbeat racing, dancing sexier than ever now. Kayleigh materialized through the fog to Bauhaus' *'Kick in the Eye'*...

"KAYLEIGH! You weren't lying, the Ladies' is *sooo* much fun...it's mental in there...this woman gave me some... and Se – *someone* snogged me, and he was, like, *the* best kisser ever and – "

"Have you seen Seb?" she cut in.

"Nah, maybe he's at the bar. Let's go an' see. I want another drink."

He kissed Kayleigh, got more vodkas in, said that as it'd be closing in forty minutes we might as well leave soon, and once we'd downed them we did – drunkenly tripping up the stairs in titters; traversing town in drunken disorder and careening arm-in-arm-in-arm with Seb-in-the-middle groping my arse; however drunk Seb was, still remembering where he'd parked and how to drive…

Outside Kayleigh's, he pecked her on the cheek and she and I tumbled out. I hugged her goodnight and took her place beside him. We'd not reached the end of her road when he pulled over.

"You ever had sex?" he asked.

"Well, I was pissed on Pernod at the school slag's house party last year an' we were under her dining-table kissing an' I was feeling her tits…I knew I was gay, but, you know… somehow she managed to get my hand in her knickers an' she had *this* much of this finger in her fanny" – I measured an inch of my middle digit – "before I realized what she was doing…DON'T LAUGH!…I nearly shat myself…it was like having my finger raped. I was already terrified of fannies from seeing them in porno mags …I was in such a rush to get away that I whacked my head on the underneath of the table jumping up…DON'T LAUGH!…it fucking hurt…an' then I – "

He cut me off with a kiss, then reeled in his tongue and teased "You're talkative, aren't you? You'll have to be quiet when we get to mine so you don't wake my parents," then hit the gas. Embarrassed into silence, I hardly breathed the rest of the ride…

Seb switched on the bedside lamp, hastily stripped then unhurriedly removed his watch, bangles and necklaces. I stood admiring his physique – musclier than I'd imagined, as smooth as mine but with dark brown pubes, as pale as mine but not pasty like me. Scared he'd go off me if he saw my gingerpubed weediness I hung fire till he was in bed and appealed, "Turn away!" My eyes were rooted on him as I undressed, burying those unsexy saggy M&S Y-fronts Mom bought me that were a graceless reminder of how childishly un-sophisticated I was beneath my outer symbols of Goth sophistication.

I dove under the duvet and lay there rigid until he rolled over and unfroze me…languorously stroking his left hand down my body…my boner spasming as he brushed past it to my thigh…across to my inner thigh then up…fondling my balls gingerly. Then he kicked off the covers, clenched the base of my cock, and went down…taunting my glans with the tip of his tongue, each gentle nuance making me shudder, nibbling it ever so gently which made me whimper, tonguing it again, then nibbling again…sinking his maw ever so gradually…lazily gliding up then down…his tongue all the while swirling round and around while his right hand caressed my flesh. I wasn't so self-conscious now, not now he, groaning as much as me, was so into me…

Seb paused. "How's that?"

"A-m-ay-z-i-n-g," I sighed, beaming ear-to-ear. "We weren't taught that in sex education!"

"Yeah, well, you never had me teachin' you, did you?!"

He top-and-tailed and there was a clumsy clash of knees, elbows and chins…Seb frowning, smirking as if to say *'sex can be awkward even if you're a pro'* before steering himself towards my nervous jaws…instructing me how…once I'd got the hang and had spent an eternity demonstrating my newfound talent, Seb reciprocating…our satisfied *whoahs* spurring the other on to suck like the survival of the species depended on it…when he began to wank and suck me simul-taneously I copied…gathering momentum and unrelenting…

Seb pulling away, panting…me pulling away just as I…
flawlessly in synch, spuming enough to float a sperm whale…

"Ugh, that was…wow, I'm sooooo happy…this has been
the best day ever…that dog in Rackhams…an' getting thrown
outta that pub…an' snogging that guy…God, I hope I don't
see him again…and us in the Zig Zag and…well, I've fancied
you since I first saw you," I waffled as I dried myself on the
t-shirt Seb had already dampened.

"And…er…I…I…I *do* really, really, really love you," I said,
snuggling up to him. He was unconscious…

Unable to sleep, the words *'thisss will keep you awake aaall
night'* looped as I watched the LED clock display creep from
4 to 5 to 6 to 7 to 8 to 9 until, my morning glory dawning, I
wondered how it would feel to screw someone. I mounted
Seb, conveniently lain facedown, spread-eagle…

"It'll need to be much harder than that if you wanna stick
it in," he mumbled unenthusiastically into the pillow. After
working it solid, attempting to bore him again, he added dryly,
"I'm really tight. You won't get it in without loadsa spit." One
single-minded dick and one hole, each slimy with saliva, all
set, I shoehorned my end in, and was about to give it the big
heave-ho when…

Seb's mom shrieked at the spectacle of an over-made-up
underage deviant, bum to the wind, sodomizing her 'straight'
son…Seb reared like *Buckaroo*, sending me careering to the
shagpile and shrouding himself in duvet like that would pull
the wool over her eyes…I scrambled for something to shield
my ardour – in three minds whether I should snort at the
slapstick aspect, or apologize to Seb's mom, or chastise her
for bursting in unannounced. But she'd withdrawn as fast as
she'd come.

"How embarrassing…God, if that'd been my mom I'd have died…it was hilarious, though, wasn't it?" I sniggered, still ravenous for that full anal breakfast and rousing myself to resume proceedings. But there'd be no fourth crack.

"C'mon, get dressed. I'll take you home," said Seb poker-faced, dressing hastily then ladling my heap of junk jewellery into my bag to hurry me along.

"You…you…you…" Seb's dad's vocabulary failed him as we crossed on the stairs – Seb snarling, "Don't start!" and not uttering another word till we arrived at mine when all he mustered was an apathetic "Nah" to my coffee invite. Not put off, I closed in for a kiss. He declined that too, muttering, "It's not cuz I don't wanna, it's just somebody might see," and pointing at Mom's car. He had a point.

"Are you gonna take my 'phone number then?" I asked.

Seb engraved it on his *B&H* pack with a spent biro. I made him recite it back to check it was readable. He swore he'd call later, and I got out – waving after his yellow Capri, on cloud nine.

Mom's nose stayed buried in *The Observer.* No "Hi", let alone a "Where have you been?" when I walked in. *Oh, so she's not talking to me again? Well, that's fine,* I thought. Because, having acquired a taste for vodka, her disregard meant she wouldn't notice me spirit hers to my bedroom. *AND I'm gonna smoke too.* Aidan smoked anyway, so if she smelt it she'd suppose it was the stale hangover from his nasty habit…

Still smeared in yesterday's make-up and stinking of sex and BO, yet super-soigné with Mom's *Smirnoff* and my *Marlboro,* I browsed my records for something suitably dirty and urbane to play, hesitating at Marc and the Mambas' double LP, *'Torment & Toreros'*. I'd only once played it in its entirety because…well, apart from the handful of foot-tappers which I'd loved straight off, and that sleazy waltz riddled with *'herpes' 'fucks' 'dick' 'whore'* and *'masturbation'* which – knowing Mom'd abhor it – I'd coerced myself to adore, the rest were turgid dirges I either didn't have patience for, or – with my limited life-experience – I just hadn't *got*. I felt worldlier today though, and it was definitely the dirtiest most sophisticated record I owned, so…

Acoustic guitars drifted in, strumming no particular melody…after a few bars the guitars picked up by piano – its tango tempo as precise as the guitars' weren't…then came boozy violins…then a tortured sax entered the fray, screeching shriller and shriller against the timpani thump-thump-thumping forth…an instrumental war of wills, then *POW!* The overture collided into a prowling stray cat strut. I merrily *miaow-oh-wow-wowed* along, and in the fade-outs between *'Boss Cat'* and cinematic chansons about matadors and crestfallen idols I sipped Mom's vodka…

> *'What you earn, heaven knows,*
> *it goes straight up your nose'*

Now I get it: cocaine!
There whumped an ominous *BAM!*

> *'I was always a lonely boy'*

confessed Marc, melancholy inching its spidery way upon my joy…I swigged some vodka…

> *'I never acted like a boy'*

74

mirrored me, Sindy dolls and princess dress-up, despising football and boys' rough-and-tumble...

> *'I noticed your eyes today,*
> *avoiding me today'*

were Seb's eyes this morning. *He's playing it cool, I know he loves me or he wouldn't have done that,* I'd thought in the car home, letting it pass, eyeballing his expert lips.

My eyes wandered from wall to wall...

> *'Thinking how lonesome I've grown,*
> *all alone in my room...'*

Until I'd met Kayleigh, these 2-D Siouxsies and Soft Cells and the Monroe and Harlow posters had been witness to my listless loneliness, and might soon be again. I swigged more vodka...

> *'So this is the big deal,*
> *the ultimate feeling'*

rued Marc of his first time, guiltiness corroding the lustre of mine...

From the silence swelled a harpsichord lacerated with sadistic Hendrix thrashes, Marc seething

> *'You forced me to love you'*

like Seb had me with his forceful kiss – this baroque'n'roll masochism submitting to a ponderous saga of car crash suicide so sombre it could drive teetotallers to drink.

I took another vodka swig then wilted on my bed...

'And the clock on the wall...'

...watching my clock's second hand tick slower than hours, slower than the song, willing myself into his psyche so he'd realise *I* was his destiny and 'phone any second to tell me Kayleigh was history...

At the phrase *'you fake the kiss'* waves of what-ifs shivered my skin. I curled up...

'A stupid fly, love's little insect...'

sucking my thumb as I did when feeling unloved and insecure, a synthetic snare drum hammering like a black heart...

'Playing'

Seb's lascivious glances over unsuspicious Kayleigh's shoulder

'Stealing the feelings'

pressing me to admit *I love you*, just to claim it with a leer

'Pushing, your icy fingers'

his pushy hands cold-heartedly groping my arse behind her back.

'Your jealous mind so disapproving'

was the look of jealousy on Seb's face, when he'd said *Don't kiss anyone else tonight* after I'd kissed that bloke.

'And encouraged my fears'

like Seb had mine by nourishing the insecurity I wore on my sleeve with his blow-by-blow boasts of older, handsomer, horse-hung conquests who weren't virgins like me.

> *'You got your revenge*
> *For the love that I lent'*

surrendered Marc to whomever.

Elegies to self-seeking eroticism and the torment of emotional manipulation reduced to embers any starry-eyed delusions I had that sex with Seb was the start of some grand amour. My eyes brimmed at the realisation I'd been just a notch on his bedpost...

What if he's at Kayleigh's telling her we did it, making out it was me who came on to him?

My tears bled as *'My Little Book of Sorrows'* recounted being bullied at school, flooding long after the overwrought climax to this torture-de-force, *'Beat Out That Rhythm On A Drum'*, had shush'd into thin air...

Too sapped to move, the stillness broken by sobs and the *pht-pht-pht* of the stylus stuck in the lock groove, I only dragged my corpse off the bed because Mom called "DINNER!" I wasn't hungry. Toying with my food, parents who weren't bothered about where their baby boy had been last night were oblivious to the tear-wrecked *No7* staining his cheeks in zebra stripes, or that he was inebriated, or...well, Mom smelt nicotine but like I'd predicted she roasted Aidan for that. Then she turned on me.

"Just eat it, will you. I didn't spend two hours slaving over a hot stove for fun. And hurry up! You stink, you need a bloody bath!"

I scrubbed myself clean of Seb, holed-up my sad self in my room, and for the next few days – other than venturing downstairs to eat or out to the offie to blow the dough the Nans had sent me on *Smirnoff* – I stayed put, replaying The Mambas' miserablest moments until Mom and Dad rolled in from a party on Christmas Eve…

"WHADDYA MEAN YOU HAVEN'T WRAPPED THE PRESENTS YET?" she thundered. "NO WONDER THE KIDS'RE SO BLOODY USELESS, THEY GET THAT FROM YOU, YOU CRETIN!"

Tearing Marc off the turntable, I stuck on that Siouxsie rant.

> *'Fuck the mothers kill the others,*
> *kill the mothers fuck the others.'*

Mom clomped upstairs, bawling "CARL! TURN THAT DISGUSTING RACKET OFF!"
Paralytic, Dad crawled after her dribbling *I-love-you's.*

"DON'T COME TO BED 'TIL THEY'RE DONE!" she issued, and slammed their bedroom door in Dad's face.

I awoke to Mom harping on at Dad for wrapping everything in their carriers. When she unpeeled one and pulled out a pair of mumsy sheepskin moccasins, she – who'd never worn any footwear with heels under three inches, not even slippers – completely let rip.
"WHAT THE HECK…IF YOU THINK I'D WEAR THESE BLOODY THINGS, YOU OBVIOUSLY STILL DON'T KNOW ME AFTER TWENTY FIVE YEARS!"

Her anger evaporated into waterworks then spiralled into a regurgitation of every grudge she held.

She doesn't stop, even on Christmas Day! She's constantly complaining but what the fuck's she got to complain about: one bad present? I fucking hate her! I wish I'd never been born. And most of the time she acts like she wishes I'd never been born either, and what kind of mother does that?

I'd be fifteen in eight days. But if my spirits were as sallow then as they were now, I wouldn't feel like celebrating the beginning of what'd undoubtedly wind up being a Kayleigh-less year in this glum slog from womb to tomb. Not that ours was a family who'd ever celebrated birthdays…

6

'Yesterdays and broken dreams that somehow slipped away...'

'Between The Lines' Janis Ian

Janet's recollections were abstract. The last thing she could remember with absolute certainty was the relief of her waters finally breaking two weeks past her December 20th due date. Her Christmas and New Year could've been ruined, but her predicament hadn't put her off wetting her unborn's head and drowning her sorrows with double-measure *Gordon's*. It had been Thursday teatime, January 2nd 1969, when John finally sped her to hospital with Aidan squealing boisterously down her lughole. She hoped she wouldn't need the overnight vanity case overloaded with the accoutrements she used to transform herself into Dusty Springfield each dawn – that the baby would slip out so quick that she'd be back by 8.45 for *The Main News* and a G'n'T, extra-light on the T.

Four hours passed.
"Push, keep it up!"
Five hours.
"You're doing brilliantly, Janet. C'mon, you can do it!"

Six....
"Push, hard as you can now. C'mon, now really push!"

Fuzzy from the pills she was still popping for the postnatal depression that hadn't abated since Aidan's birth three years ago, Janet only heard the midwife's encouragement as a tinny, hazy, distant voice. Had she had the strength she'd have walloped the midwife into 2001 because she *was* fucking well pushing: the wilful incubus just didn't want to come out. Numb below the waist from epidural, disconnected physically and mentally, she began to convulse…

Seven hours.
"Please stay calm – for you and the baby," urged the obstetrician to no avail.

Eight…
Pained yelps as the epidural wore off, her normally pristine platinum bouffant a sweat-ravaged thatch, she was on the homestretch…

The instant the umbilical cord was cut the turbulent patient was injected with sedatives, out for the count before she'd even held her newborn, insensible to the healthy 9lb bundle of joy being cleaned of placenta only feet away. And, just like the first time round – when John thought he'd fulfilled his spousal duty by fertilising her eggs and didn't need to stick around to witness the phenomenon of childbirth – he wasn't there to hold her hand this time either. Telling himself it was pointless three people suffering, he'd taken Aidan home hours ago. As the doctor read Janet's medical report, his main concern was her state of mind. While the baby was being swaddled in terry-towelling, he telephoned Mr Stanley to advise he sanction electroconvulsive therapy on his heavily sedated spouse's behalf. If hundred-volt short sharp shocks were what the doctor ordered, that was fine with John. He agreed immediately. Anything to stop Janet's erratic behaviour…

"Oh, and by the way, Mr Stanley. Congratulations! It's a girl!"

So, while his wife fried in Psychiatric and his daughter desperately bawled for contact in Maternity, as hanging around hospital with a tetchy toddler would've been no fun, John took Aidan to the cinema to see *Chitty Chitty Bang Bang*. But he wasn't totally uninvolved with the daughter he'd yet to meet. Singing along to *'Truly Scrumptious'* he did manage to think up a name: Caroline.

When nurses broke it to him that Caroline had a penis, that the doctor had made a cock-up, he shrugged. They'd call her Carl instead.

On being confronted with her squawking son, Janet had an even greater shock than she did acquainting her Jackson Pollock brain to the bombshell that she'd undergone ECT.

"Christ, he's ugly! He looks like a bloomin' rat...and he's so bloody noisy."

If she'd been too incapacitated to cradle him previously, now she hadn't the inclination – especially as his abundant jet curls were inherited from a busybody mother-in-law she couldn't abide. Janet prayed that was *all* he'd inherit from John's side, because heaven help Carl if he grew up to be the slightest bit like her father-in-law.

Everybody who'd ever had the bad luck to meet Jack Stanley agreed he was the grumpiest, most unpleasant person they'd ever met – the chip on his shoulder stemming from having a slovenly mother who only lived to Charleston, added to by slicing off his own thumb at seventeen, and topped off by being bald at the age of twenty. Not that her parents were much better than the Stanleys...

Winnie had elevated doing nothing – except spending inordinate hours at 'Hair by Jean', equal testimony both to Winnie's skill at sitting still and Jean's expertise at relentlessly reinventing the wash–rollerset-and-blowout to appease flighty Winnie – to a high art. It was as though she'd only had the girls to be her handmaids, although it always seemed to first-born Janet that she did more skivvying than Winnie's golden girl Linda. And when their dad Billy wasn't at his allotment, his diversion from the abrasive reality of a dreary factory job in Smethwick, a black-soot suburb a stone's throw from the city's splendid shrines to imperialist glories, he spent his waking hours at the pub. With scant attention from either parent, bonny Janet, Soho Street's May Queen of 1953, sought solace in books. She sailed her eleven plus; she got six O-levels; and she was three years into the five-year engineer apprenticeship which would lead to a wage-packet visa out of this loveless home – two claustrophobic rooms above a grocer's shop that rang with her mom and dad's constant silences, even more unbearable after the arrival of the two brothers Janet was a proxy mother to – when she decided that accepting her first-love John's engagement ring would mean a speedier escape…

Like fifty million others who anticipated the arrival of a colourful era to eradicate the post-war austerity which had shadowed '50s grey Britain, Janet had been optimistic about the '60s. She'd begun the decade with a trip up the aisle. But within months of getting married, she realised she might've made an awful gaffe. John might be handsome and a good lover, kind and funny and an ambitious grafter set on starting his own electrical firm, a man who'd provide for their off-spring should they have any, but he'd never stimulate a woman of her intelligence. Before six months were up she considered leaving him, had even gone as far as viewing bedsits, but she chickened out…

They worked their knuckles to the bone till they saved the deposit for a house; they ground their bones till they could afford to inch up the property ladder; and although motherhood wasn't really on her agenda, missing her period was grounds for celebration. Life had been peachy until those baby blues had kicked-in. Too late to turn back the hands of a biological clock she'd never felt tick, at least she knew there'd be no more happy accidents thanks to The Pill.

God, how could John have so blithely consented to Electric Shock Therapy?! Didn't it enter his pea-brain that her malaise had been multiplied by his failure to be the hands-on paterfamilias she needed, by her aborted career ambitions, and by that tenacious spermatozoon which had thrown pre-natal depression into the equation and further multiplied her malaise? Watching the moon landing on telly, she thought they might as well have sent *him* up into space because he was already on another planet to her!

John was at work. Aidan was at school. Carl – whose raven curls had turned ginger – was caterwauling upstairs, and Janet was sat at the kitchen table mopping her forlorn mascara on an already soggy hankie. She leapt up to attack a radio *ooh-ooh-ooh-ing* the intro to *'Baby Love'* on some retro chart rundown – that was the last bloody song she wanted to hear right now – and thumped the off button. Her Swinging Sixties hadn't been so swinging after all. God, where did the last eighteen months go? It was 1971! She'd *have* to stir herself out of this non-existence and regain her *oomph* or she'd go doolally. She had needs, for fuck's sake! For starters, she'd get her Fallopian tubes tied. She liked sex too much to keep her legs crossed forever, she couldn't rely on contraceptive tablets, and she daren't depend on *Durex* and crossing her fingers. And her peroxide pile-up was a vestige of unhappier times which needed modernising if she were to contemplate some new vocation. Struth knows what she'd do though, because technological advances excluded a return to engineering...

"I'm going out...*alone*. It won't kill you to look after *your* kids for once, will it?"

Her sarcastic tenor dared John to concoct an excuse, but she was gone before he had chance to think of one.

At the hairdressers, with her transformation in progress, Janet discouraged chitchat by opening her *Guardian* – the point of flying solo today had been to have some 'me time', after all – avidly reading an article about the Department of Education crying out for applicants. Apparently, there was a crippling deficit of teachers, the state of affairs so critical that training wasn't mandatory – providing applicants were qualified in whatever area they applied to teach. Teaching hadn't occurred to her.

"Is there a *Solihull News* anywhere?" she asked.

Jacqui *had* seen one; she'd find it while Janet's colour was being washed.

Back from the basin, Janet flicked straight to 'Sits Vac' and there it was:

'Metalwork and/or Technical Drawing teacher urgently required. Experienced teachers and those seeking first appointment welcome. The successful applicant will have qualification and/or relevant work experience in engineering. All enquiries to...'

Fate! With her credentials, including 1963's *Apprentice of the Year* at GKN Screws & Fasteners Ltd, she was the ideal candidate. Wet hair or no wet hair, this was a golden opportunity not to be missed! She ran to the front desk to make that all-important call. *'Yes, the situation is still vacant. Can you come in today at 3 o'clock, Mrs Stanley?'*

Jacqui finished blow-drying Janet's honey-blonde Hanoi Jane feather-cut and sprayed it 'til there was no way a single strand would fly away. With an hour to kill, unhindered by the pushchair she sometimes wanted to push – cargo and all – under a moving car, without a bored Aidan bleating *'I'm bored'* whilst she tried on clothes, Janet celebrated her freedom and cat-walked half of Richard Shops' stock around the changing-room until she found something with that wow-factor to wow her prospective employer: a khaki safari-style shirt-dress. A shoe-shop pit-stop to assure she was top-to-toe height-of-fashion, best six-inch cork-wedge platform forward, she stepped confidently into the 'Me Decade'…

Selling herself to her potential boss, glossing over the depressing gap in her résumé by fibbing "Those five years were devoted to raising my sons," Janet's confidence soared when he said, "You're definitely right for this post." She was taken aback as he continued, "With start of term two months away, quite frankly we're desperate." She relaxed when he added, "Checking references will just be a formality," supremely confident that she'd pass the "…probationary period to assess your ability in the classroom". As he rounded-off the meeting with "Welcome to Secondary Modern Education, Mrs Stanley," Janet was jubilant. She'd done it! She'd got the job! She couldn't wait to tell John…

His car's not there, nice he's taking fatherhood seriously and taken the boys out. Great, a bit more me-time, she thought on arriving home. But, turning the key, Janet saw what looked like blood stains on the porch tiles – a bloody trajectory leading through the hall to a…*What the?!*…mound of bloodied towels in the lounge. Horrified, Janet knocked-up the neighbours, but no-one at 20 or 24 could shed any light on the goings on at no.22 – although they were as alarmed as her once they saw the gory scene. Hysterical, Janet made 'phone calls to everyone in her address book too. Just as she was about to call 999, John waltzed in carrying Carl, with grouchy Aidan at his side…

John's chipper "Did you have a nice day while I took care of the kids, love?" – as if neither the bloodbath which had greeted her nor Carl's bandaged head were causes for concern – triggered her to explode. "WHADDYA MEAN *WHILE I TOOK CARE OF THE KIDS?!* FROM WHAT I CAN SEE, YOU'VE BEEN BLOODY USELESS! WHAT THE HELL HAPPENED?"

Knowing she'd get more satisfaction from an infant too guileless to cook up fictions, shushing John, she repeated the question to Aidan.

"Dad said he had to go to work and after he left Carl started running 'round the house playing aeroplanes and I told him to stop but he wouldn't and he fell and smashed his head on the fireplace and it started bleeding and I wrapped it in towels because it was bleeding a lot and I got him his teddy and Dad screamed when he got back," spewed Aidan in one breath.

"So something was *that* urgent that you thought it'd be okay to leave *Aidan* in charge?!"

"I didn't think you'd be gone so long. Where were you?" countered John, setting down the injured infant who toddled towards his irate mother for comfort which never came.

"Don't turn this around on me! And I don't need to answer to you…haven't you heard of women's lib? But for *your*

information, while I was in Raymonds having my hair done…
and you haven't even *commented* on it……shush, it's too late
for compliments now… I SAID SHUSH! I saw a teaching
vacancy in the paper. I rang the school and they asked me
to come for an interview, and I tried calling to tell you I'd be
late but I suppose you were already in Casualty…SHUT UP!
I'M TALKING! And I got the bloody job…don't try changin'
the subject by congratulating me! And what kind of welcome's
this?" roared Janet, pointing at the congealed splodges. "And
you couldn't even be arsed to leave a bloody note! Well,
you can clean the bloody carpet 'cause I'm damned if I'm doin'
it! I'm telling you now, things are going to change 'round here
or else!"

She retreated to the kitchen and read another chapter of
The Female Eunuch, growing a little more emancipated with
each paragraph of Germaine Greer's radical manifesto; John
spent hours up to his elbows in soapy water, emasculated by
pinker-by-the-minute suds; Aidan bounded upstairs to play
with his *Action Man*; and Carl's mind was occupied with something other than a squidgy nappy or his empty tum which had
been life's most pressing issues up to now: trying to scratch
those itchy stitches that had made his mom so mad.

Now that she'd discovered her rage, Janet used it on John
frequently. Whenever she did, Aidan would make himself
scarce for fear that she'd direct it at him, and Carl would rub
his head, confused about what he'd done to cause it this time
when there were no stitches there to scratch.

Things didn't change…

"Did you have a nice day, love?" chirped John, breezing in
late again to yet another charred meal without an apology.

"Well, if you consider the battle I had force-feeding Carl his cornflakes, and dealing with him kicking off about getting dressed…God, it hurt *me* smacking him more than it hurt him!… and playing up when I left him at the child-minder's this morning, then even worse when I collected him this afternoon because he didn't want to leave, then doing his disappearing act again in Sainsbury's, then letting the bloody budgie out of its cage and managing to open a window, and the ruckus I had to contend with when the damn thing flew away…oh, *and* six and a half hours teaching teenagers when half of them don't want to learn…then yes, I've had a *very nice day,* thank-you."

"That's nice," replied John, sawing through his incinerated sirloin.

"WHADDYA MEAN *'THAT'S NICE'?* DON'T YOU LISTEN TO A BLOODY WORD I SAY? YOU DON'T KNOW WHAT A HANDFUL CARL IS!"

"Aw, he'll calm down once he starts playgroup. As soon as he's around lads his own age he'll see it's not normal to want to play with dolls or wear your wedding dress," reasoned John like he was suddenly the expert on parenting.

Carl so loathed the idea of having to interact with other children that on day one he'd insured none would ever venture within ten yards of him by fighting a girl over a frock from the dressing-up box, then slapping some lad who'd giggled at him for slipping it on; he'd stuck his tongue out at the supervisor for daring to say boys didn't wear dresses, wriggling free when she'd tried to disrobe him and hitching-up his skirt and running away screaming; John got so much grief when he attempted to coax Carl's Y chromosome with a *Tonka Toy* on a Saturday outing that the only way to shut him up was to buy him the *Sindy* he wouldn't let go of; he'd taken his son on a one-off supermarket shop, and having experienced what Janet had to cope with weekly – Carl dashing off into the arms of an employee and reporting himself lost so he'd hear his name over the tannoy – he'd sworn he wouldn't be doing that again; instead, reeking of oil and unapologetic, John habitually returned home late from the factory to hundreds more ruined dinners.

Janet frowned at the bridal gown Carl had only abandoned because its train had got so mangled by his bicycle-chain that the prissy boy wouldn't be seen dead in it anymore. Gathering up the silk heap from the veranda floor, she thought about her dad's words in the limousine on their way to church on what should have been the happiest day of her life: *It's not too late to change your mind, Jan.* Billy had repeated them to the beat of Wagner's *Wedding March* as he led her up the aisle; he'd whispered them in her ear at the altar; and if she'd had a crystal ball to foretell how little John would follow 'love, honour and obey' she'd have probably listened…

She squashed her wedding weeds into the bin; sympathetic though she was with strikers protesting over the Conservative government's pay caps, if the bin-men's strike spread to Solihull before *hers* was emptied and she had to face the wretched thing for as long as it lasted, then her sympathies might turn from staunch socialist to Tory. Fortunately the strike didn't, so her principles were safe. From the kitchen window she watched the dress get gobbled-up with the street's garbage, twisting at her gold band as the truck rolled away, rueing that marriage couldn't be so easily disposed of, not when there were kids…

To whitewash over her disillusionment she wed herself to her profession and redistribution of its financial rewards, taking on the headmaster's challenge of teaching Maths with such aplomb that her pupils' O-level pass rates were superlative; taking a giant leap up the property ladder; blotting out the depression which blighted her nights with a bouncy new hairdo, fur coats, *Enny* handbags to match every outfit and a bottle-green 'R'-reg *MGB GT V8*; and moving to a new job as a college lecturer where new colleagues broadened her horizons…

"I'm organising an outing to Greenham Common. Do you fancy it?" asked a flat-shod activist co-worker.

"Count me in!" answered Janet, chomping at the bit to explore pastures anew, and in her spare minutes she re-read her Germaine Greer in earnest…

As she protested against nuclear weapons, wielding her CND placard knee-deep in mud and adding her high-decibel soprano to a chant set to *'Frère Jacques'*:

> *We are women, we are women,*
> *We are strong, we are strong,*
> *We say no, we say no,*
> *To the bomb, to the bomb*

as she wrestled her way onto the frontline of those militants endeavouring to invade the RAF base and was manhandled by misogynist riot police menacing "BACK OFF YOU DYKE, OR WE'LL ARREST YOU!" – and arrest and a few days in prison would've been respite from domestic obligations, except regrettably she wasn't – the exhilaration she felt being at Greenham felt like she'd leapt off Navajo Point and into the Grand Canyon to discover she could fly. *This* was what the Swinging Sixties must've been like: anti-Vietnam War demos, sit-ins, *'Give Peace a Chance'*… Janet was having a blast. Right up until the moment one hirsute pair of dungarees had the balls to denunciate her, as immaculately dolled-up as ever, of "titivating yourself for the enemy, you traitor!"

Her boorish brother-in-law may have ridiculed, *'Are you gonna turn lesbian too?'* when she'd said she was off to Greenham; and her record collection might include a Janis Ian and a Joan Armatrading; but if *Coty Shimmer* and *Carmen* heated rollers were verboten by misandrists who'd literally castrated 'men' from 'women' to create 'wimmin' in *Spare Rib* magazine, well, *she* wouldn't be quaffing from the furry cup anytime soon...

"Piss off! I'm a wife *and* a mother, *and* I work full-time. I'm more feminist than you," Janet growled at her accuser, internalizing *As long as I'm Mrs John Stanley I won't ever be properly liberated though.* Despite her Leftie beliefs, she was won over by an orator rallying, "We owe it to our suffragette foresisters to vote Conservative at the next election! Only a woman Prime Minister can bring wider opportunities for the sisterhood, for us, for all 'wimmin'!"

Janet mightn't be able to drop everything and join those professional protestors who were plotting the setting up of a permanent Women's Peace Camp – for one thing, where would she plug in her curlers? But the ideas she'd heard that day had planted the seeds of her own feminist initiative...

"There's a hole in the prospectus," she told the college's head of HR. "I've come up with a course targeted specifically at introducing women...or reintroducing those who've been out of the loop...you know, bringing up families and so on...to traditionally male spheres like engineering or plastering or plumbing...help them gain confidence, arrange visits to employers, get work-experience placements…call it *Wider Opportunities for Women, WOW* for short."

"It sounds great, especially in today's climate. If you can take on the extra workload you've got my backing. I hope it doesn't end up 'Opportunities for Wider Women' though, because those Women's Libbers aren't all as pretty as you, Jan," he said. Only if he'd chased her 'round his office pinching her bum to the *Benny Hill* theme could he have been more patronizing…

WOW was clearly what women of all sizes and from all walks of life wanted because on Open Day they swamped her stand. She sold it so successfully that inside an hour it was fully subscribed. Now her boys were nine and eleven and plenty capable of overseeing themselves for the odd hour or five, she used the summer recess – and her feminine wiles – to woo businesses. There was such overwhelming interest that *WOW* would have wings to soar well into the '80s too. Its success drew the attention of regional TV producers who dispatched a film crew to interview the project's initiator for *ATV Today*, the 6 o'clock news show.

Gathered 'round the box with the kids whining through the tedious bits, *'When you gonna be on?'* at long last the anchorman heralded, *'Earlier, Anne Diamond met an enterprising lady who's making waves…'*

The fizzy brunette on TV might be engrossed in Mom's treatise on female equality; and a hundred thousand viewers might see this former engineer and working mum and *'inspiration to every woman watching'* as Superwoman; but she was still that same lunatic who'd whack us, shout, pack her suitcase and walk out on us once in a while, and who'd lob plates at Dad, who might have to dodge another one later for missing her fifteen minutes of fame.

With her career in full summer Janet even fooled herself she was happy sometimes, but despite her smokescreen, with John as unsupportive as unset blancmange, blacklisted by her doctor from receiving anti-depressants in 1976, beneath her veneer there festered a wintery discontent which even the sunniest days couldn't entirely thaw...

7

'Sexcrime, sexcrime, nineteen eighty-four...'

'*Sexcrime*' Eurythmics

Kayleigh was her usual cheery self when I telephoned her after a truly miserable Christmas to ask was she still up for giving me a Mohican like she'd said she would at The Zig Zag – and when I got to hers, she hugged me warmly, sticking on the 12" of Culture Club's '*Victims*' and cooing all lovey-dovey, "Seb bought it me, he says it's our tune, that line *Push aside those that whisper never*". He obviously hadn't betrayed our infidelity…

"You're quiet, is everythin' alright?" she quizzed, razor-in-hand. Not the safest time to let slip that *she* was the victim with an unfaithful boyfriend, a sword-swallower who'd swallowed mine, I lied "I'm fine," and side-tracked her with "I can't wait for Louch's reaction to this!"

By 8.55am, Louch had quarantined his sickest inmate in First Aid again. The peripatetic optician had tested me in here last term, and the evil bitch had diagnosed severe myopia, but as jam-jar bins wouldn't have sat well atop panda eyes, and knowing full well that Mommy Dearest would've relished the opportunity to make me look a numpty, I'd instantly binned it. As I squinted at the blurry eye-chart, sure the problem was tipsiness from three too many pre-school tipples, not short-sightedness, it was impossible to focus on quadratic equations. Instead I worried whether Kayleigh hadn't returned my last three calls because she *had* found out. I was dreading seeing Kayleigh at break but it didn't happen. So grave was Louch's concern that my condition might contaminate his school that he kept me in solitary confinement all day – his petrified secretary scuttling in at midday to throw down a tray of food, and again at home-time to hand at arm's length an envelope addressed 'Mrs Stanley'.

Mom was in the laundry-room doing her ironing. I left the letter on the breakfast bar, went upstairs, and promptly forgot about it. There were bigger fish to fry: like who'd maintain my Mohican should Kayleigh and I fall out? And should I add colour to my make-up? And would it be wrong to bang a quickie out over that heart-breaking, two-timing tosser Seb? And why did Kayleigh think Bananarama were crap just because they didn't give a fuck? They *were* ex-Punks, and if their fingers-up ethos wasn't pure Punk, what was? As the 'Nana's platter *Deep Sea Skiving* swept over me, having conceded that Seb was *still* sexy as hell, I'd just unzipped my flies when an almighty "WHAAAGH!!" quaked the house to its foundations.

Mom stormed in waving Louch's missive.

"He's suspending you for – and I quote – *antisocial activities!*"

"I *was* antisocial, he locked me in the First Aid room for seven hours, didn't even let me out to go to the loo."

"WHAT? That's illegal! And he goes on... *If Carl continues to wear this obscene hairstyle, I will have no option but to expel him!*"

I should be so lucky. Seeing as mom would be at school pulverising Louch first thing, it would be my misfortune to be on time for Fag Ash Lil's Physics yawn-a-thon…

"Black hair dye didn't affect his grades *or* his conduct did it? He's had a Mohican, not a lobotomy," said Mom.

"Didn't you receive my letter informing you that Carl is on report for truancy?"

Bastard snitch, it's not my fault I got caught, it's yours.

PE had always been torture, and – fed up of being wet-towel-whipped in the showers – I'd elected that games could take a running jump. Mr Mellor didn't give a toss if I played hookey if it saved him the hassle of refereeing fifty pricks spitting *Watch your arses, there's a shirt-lifter about*, but Louch had spoilt this mutually beneficial arrangement by covering one week when Mellor was ill, and had put me on report just as autumn fell.

"The way you victimise him it's no wonder he skives. You'll need more ammunition than that, you are *NOT* gonna jeopardise his chances. He's already halfway through his O-level coursework…anyway, I'm too busy to find another school so he's staying, understood?"

Louch nodded servilely.

"Good," said Mom, tossing his letter in the waste paper basket on her way out…

That morning break, the knuckle-dragging Thin Knot who gave me most abuse rammed his spotty mug in my face and cussed "Fuckin' cocksucker!" as he sauntered by.

"YEAH I AM, AN' I LOVE IT!"

"WHOSE COCK HAVE *YOU* SUCKED, HALES'S?" he responded, referring to our effete music teacher.

"NO, HIS NAME'S SEB AND HIS COCK'S TWICE THE SIZE OF YOURS!"

Scott bombed at me, bidding "SUCK THIS!"

Before I could duck his fist landed square on my chin and knocked me for six, my skull heaping injury on injury as it spanked the melamine. Star-blind, I saw Mr Whittell come into focus past the rapt bystanders. I faltered over...

"Fight your own battles, you puffta," muttered Whittell.

Right then, I copped Louch, stood cross-armed, watching. Hoping he'd do the headmasterly thing and act without prejudice I headed towards him. Shaking his head, leering a *Scott-deserves-a-prize-and-Mr-Whittell-deserves-a-promotion* smile he made for his office. I went after him but he slammed the door – his renunciation activating laughter which rapidly ascended to gay-baiting...not just the Thin Knots but some who'd never coo *boo* to a goose too...a feral free-for-all...the braying horde, clanging and maddening, hemming me into a corner, atremble and wanting to cry. Instead, frailty tipped me to flip, "I FUCKIN' HATE THIS FUCKIN' SHITHOLE! YOU'RE ALL FUCKIN' WANKERS!"

Shocked into silence, they froze at once. Although what should've made me feel triumphant left me feeling as exposed as Solihull's resident nutter must have when she'd come-on in McDonalds wearing white jeans and had been laughed at in her misery and brought the place to a standstill with her fuck-heavy freak-out.

Unaware Louch had snuck out from his lair until he subpoenaed, "STANLEY, MY OFFICE NOW!" I yelled "GO AN' FUCK YOURSELF, YOU C-U-U-U-U-U-N-T!"

I bulled through the flabbergasted mob, and nearly mowed down Kayleigh, who severed our friendship with a lachrymose head-shake then sloped away shrunken-shouldered. I fled outdoors, scampering here-and-there, dithering *Where to?* when all I really wanted was to be anyplace but here, frustrated I couldn't do a bunk as *that* would offer Louch *bona fide* reason to get on the blower to Mom – if he hadn't already – to grass I'd used the 'C' word. My mind was all over the place like a madwoman's custard. *What if he overheard I sucked Seb's cock?* He'd most likely spilt *that* too, the fallout of which didn't bear contemplating. Seeking sanctuary, I decided behind the bike sheds was my best bet, so I darted there, startling smokers who cursed me for being me and not a teacher when my whirl-wind invasion caused them to chuck their half-smoked ciggies. Then the bell rang and they obediently split.

Alone at last, slumping to my knees, I burst into tears. Dejected, I felt suicidal. Overhead, branches were creaking in the wind... If hanging was good enough for Ian Curtis it was good enough for me... Untying my tie and fashioning a noose, quickly reconsidering *Climbing a tree'll ruin my nails though, an' I'd rather die than be found dead with chipped nail varnish,* I lit a fag and deliberated other avenues... *Overdose?* I remembered Lupe Vélez, the '40s movie star who'd been found with her head down the toilet covered in her own vomit. *I suppose I could shoot myself? Dunno where sells guns though. Jump under a train? Drown? Fuck that, I'd rather live an' make the whole fucking world suffer...* Not weeping any longer, I flung my butt away and headed for English, psyching myself up for a rollocking from punctuality-mad Rent-a-Tent for turning up late. Remarkably I didn't get one.

Mom didn't rollock me either, so it appeared that Louch hadn't rung her. *He still might though. I'll get my side of the story in first,* I thought – today's show of support, her talk of victimisation, and her animosity to Louch making me triply sure she'd be so outraged she'd be up there tomorrow to read him the riot act. No such luck. She pretty much parroted Whittell, and cranked up *Radio 4* to reiterate that her priority wasn't me.

Long-term, her indifference would prove more advantageous than not: as the months went by there wasn't a peep about my coming in at dawn every Sunday; not a peep about my evermore *outré* appearance; no hows-or-wheres about the sackfuls of make-up or brazenly pilfered rolls of fabric which were fundamental to modify my image week in week out were I to compete with clubland's chameleon A-listers...

It had been a restrained Saturday's thieving so far: three Roxy Music LPs and this new American singer's imaginatively titled debut album *'Madonna'* courtesy of HMV, and eight chunky bracelets and an 'Iron Lady' gunmetal-mauve lippy from Miss Selfridge. I'd gone to Rackhams' café and seen Seb and his latest buxom flame sat with some greenhorn who reminded me of last year's me, but I'd had no desire to watch what might've been the prelude to *his 'Torment & Toreros'* so I scooted before Seb saw me, down to level G to palm some white eye-pencils with which I planned to rewrite eyebrow history that night. *Nobody* had done white eyebrows yet. To confuse the security cameras I wove a convoluted exit via the handbags and hosiery and china departments, pulse accelerating as it always did at the slender likelihood of capture, now freedom was a footstep over the threshold, now I'd incontestably gotten away with it again, arrogance lifting a grin...

A hand on my shoulder wrung my entrails. A faceless voice drilled, "Don't run or I'll radio for back-up. Turn around and walk ahead, go where I tell you."

I'd had my suspicions she'd been following me but strangers regularly would, often asking inanities like

Why do you dress like that?

or

Does your mom know you wear make-up?

And occasionally they'd snap my photo, and sometimes ask for autographs which I'd dedicate **Love Stan, who doesn't! XXX** – one fossilised autograph-hunter indecently assaulting me and apologising, *Sorry duck, I had to check if you had bosoms or if you were a man. It's confusing for us oldies. It ain't like when I was young; you can't tell who's what nowadays. I do love that Boy George though, he's so comical! I prefer a nice cuppa tea to sex, too!* then bursting into a chorus of *'Karma Chameleon'*.

Rackhams' ritzy shop floor became dingy passages. On my entering security control, the surveillance hawk tore himself from a bank of monochrome monitors and spun in his swivel-chair to gawk at the real me in all my Technicolor brilliance.

"Shouldn't you be watching for shoplifters?" I sassed, and back he swivelled to his screens.

Rearranging her sari, the store detective ordered me to lay my contraband on the table. She didn't believe my lie – "I haven't stolen anythin' else" – searching my handbag and pulling out amongst other things a slightly scuffed Miss Selfridge lipstick, then peeking in my HMV carrier.

"Can I go now?"

Telephone receiver to her ear, she ignored me.

"Hello, Sarge. You'll love this one…erm, male…Caucasian…fifteen…seven eyeliners."

The gallant PC assisting me onto the van calmed my fears about incarceration, telling me "We've reserved a delightful room especially for you."

But I still didn't fancy going. I hadn't robbed Boots yet.

"My uncle was a policeman," I said, expecting dispensation.

"Good for him. Did he give it up for a life of crime?"

"No, he died."

"That's a shame, he'd be very proud his nephew's got a criminal record. Right, on your marks, get set, *GO!*"

With that, the driver crunched into top gear, burning the tarmac, siren afire, like they were transporting some sociopath society needed urgent protection from...

Particulars recorded, fingerprinted and photographed, the spray-on jeans I had on underneath my vicious-pink ballgown were frisked for lethal weapons, I was stripped of my jewellery, and then shown to a frigid cell whose only feature was an inbuilt concrete ledge hard-furnished with a prostrate skank where cushions would've been preferable.

"Here's some female company for you," the PC said. Skank's dumb response was to scowl at me like he'd rape *me* to punish the copper, if he didn't slay me first. The Thin Knots were pussies by comparison...

"Make yourself comfortable, you might be here awhile depending on how long your parents take to get here," said the PC. I tried persuading him Mom – because it would be her who'd come, not Dad – was a psycho *I* urgently needed protecting from, but he wasn't interested and clanked the cell-door.

Not the slayer I'd feared, Skank shuffled his Nikes up the bench to make space for me to sit, and tweaked his baseball cap to mask his face to indicate he didn't want to communicate. Indeterminable minutes slunk into hours. Sizing him up out of utter boredom, musing *It's weird what prison does 'cause I wouldn't look twice at him on the outside,* regretting he wasn't doing me as he was pretty hot actually, that scenario was pricked by an obtrusive clank and I was signed over to the protection of an anything-but-protective-looking Mom…

Enraged they'd let me off with a measly caution, she passed her own verdict: confiscation of all cosmetics for a month.

"That's a bit harsh. I should've murdered five kids 'cause even Myra Hindley's allowed to keep her make-up!"

"RIGHT, NOW YOU'RE GROUNDED FOR A MONTH TOO! What the hell did I do to deserve a son like you? TOO BLOODY SOFT, THAT'S WHAT! Yes, you've had it too bloody cushy, that's your problem. I never stole *anything* in my life and *we* were poor! We were lucky if we got sixpence pocket money! *And* we had to do all the chores for that because *our* mom was too bloody lazy to do them even though she didn't work! *And* we had no bathroom; *we* had a tin bath we had to fetch in from the yard once a week *and* we all had to share the water …"

I'd heard her Dickensian tale before, and tuned out.

One laborious month later, I'd finally re-written eyebrow history, and was at The Zig Zag bar, chinwagging to Wolverhampton Mark – who *hadn't* brushed me off to shove his rabidly hetero tongue down some girl's throat as was his wont – complimenting his fingernail necklace.

"Cheers Stan. I made it myself. It took years savin' up my clippings," he boasted, saying *sotto voce* "You can give us a pearl one if you wanna."

He explained what a pearl necklace was; I called him a cock-tease.

"I've gotta litre of vodka an' a pack of ready rolled joints in my car. Wanna come?"

We cruised for an idyllic age, toking on spliff after spliff, shots straight from the bottle, surround-sound saturating us in *'Faith'* by The Cure, a faultless soundscape as desolate as rainy Birmingham at 3am, as monolithic as the metropolis, as sober as I wasn't...but nicely drunk...and super stoned, tripping on transient city lights, fantastic art, the lineal precision of Mondrian's *'Broadway Boogie-Woogie'* warping into Pollock chaos, diffusing into Monet lilies as the rain fell heavier...the stereo automatic, side two... no chat but comfortably so....

Then, tension at a red light, a police car beside us, the swiftest comedown, uncomfortable silence...amber, green, indecision as to who goes first...headlights tailing us, us hanging a left, them straight on, panic over....

"Light another joint, pass us the bottle," said Mark.

...bright lights fading, in a derelict outskirt...

"Don't hog the joint, Stan!"

...decelerating to a snail's pace, he investigated side streets...

What's he looking for?

"That looks like a dead-end."

...reversing into an alley too narrow to open the doors...

How the fuck will I escape if he tries to murder me?

...killing the motor, pitch-black, just the dashboard lights...

"No-one'll disturb us here," he grinned.

Now I'm really shitting myself!

Sat for an age, no chat, vodka mutely swapping hands, I saw the *News of the World* headline: **TEEN PRE-OP SEX-SWOP GETS CHOP B4 CHOP**, an inglorious epitaph, lurid and inaccurate. The Cure clicked back to side one, sounding horribly funereal now, his knee jigging agitatedly, cracking his knuckles…

He's gonna strangle me!

…still wordless, an eternal preamble to what I prayed would be quick…

'And quickly changed the tune', commentated Robert Smith through the speakers…

"Can I kiss you, Stan?"

He did: a prolonged peck, no tongues…more vodka and another joint, me too shell-shocked to converse because *this* was Wolverhampton Mark, Jack the Lad extraordinaire, him not conversing either, no justification…then he took off that fragile necklace and hung it over the rear-view mirror, and actions spoke louder, kissing me again, tongues this time…

'Another perfect lie is choked'

…a very gay hand journeying up my petticoats, grappling to undo my spandex jeans…

'commit the sin, commit yourself'

…a very straight voice, all oily foreman, ordering "Tip your seat back an' take 'em off," him undressing too…

'caress the sounds'

…enthusiastic slurps…

'textures coat my skin'

…unaccustomed to hairy chests, curious, patting his

tentatively at first in case it would deflate me, it drove me stiffer than a pillar.

He slurped fiercer, his bobbing head and our arms tangled in an erotic game of Twister – him supporting himself with one palm on my headrest and one on the floor between my feet, my left hand mangling that virile pelt and my right cack-handedly jacking-off his donkey of a dick which was frustratingly embedded in a valley of his thighs and bent torso…more and more turned on, my breaths shorter, Mark taking his hand off the floor to engage it with his mouth…

"I think I'm gonna…"
…just his hand now, 100mph…

'See you writhe' sang Robert Smith.

…Mark's neck distended and expectant, as I adorned his collarbone his very straight voice exulting, "Yeah, oh yeah, oh yeah!"…once he'd extorted every last pearl he flopped onto his back and flogged his log two-fisted and furious, levitating his hips to spray his own neck, very gay fingertips steeping themselves in that two-tiered necklace, that nuts-and-bolts voice saying "Light us a joint"… *'Faith'* looping back to side two…

"Are you goin' to The Ku tonight, Stan?"
"Can't, I've gotta do my homework or my mom'll ground me."
"Homework – how old're you?!"
"Sixteen in six months…"

"Jailbait," he said, aghast, chuckling, trading me the vodka for the joint. "Way past your beddy-byes, isn't it, little boy? I oughta drive you home to mommy an' daddy."

"Condescending cunt, you're not drivin' us anywhere! Not 'til I've had another go on that thing! Then you can buy me a Big Mac an' large fries 'cause I'm starving, then you can take us to The Barrel Organ 'cause I want a couple of pints and I wanna see this barman, Chris, I fancy who works there. Then you can drive me home. Okay?"

"Yes Sir," saluted Mark – that two-hander, as compliant to commands as him, dutifully bouncing in salute too. Like any honourable bigmouth would do, braced for oral hara-kiri, I threw myself upon it…

I trolled-in on Mom, dismembering a roast *Chukie Chicken*, bones-and-all, with her *Moulinex* carver. She cold-shouldered me, summonsed "DINNER!" and loaded the hostess trolley, shunting it into my ankles and wheeling it over my toes, which would have hurt more if I weren't reeling from other injuries: overall bruises from going at it hell-for-leather in the confines of a 3-door hatchback Metro; the ring-sting of a bumhole gaping like it was harbouring an HGV tyre – the result of what was technically rape due to my desperation to lose my cherry despite Mark not being fussed whether he shagged me or not; penile friction burns – the upshot of what was also technically rape when Mark had imposed his pinhole virginity on me, his muscular voice demanding "Fuck us harder!" such an aphrodisiac that I couldn't pound hard enough; an almost dislocated jaw and swollen lips; not to mention tonsils raw from tens of joints…

She small-talked to Dad and Aidan but steadfastly blanked me. As I piled my plate high, I was cataloguing every uncovered crime – fag butts and *Smirnoff* in my closet; that I'd hawked my clarinet; that I'd lately begun to redistribute their wealth by relieving them of money – when Dad casually outed me.

"Aidan tells us you're gay."
O-H…M-Y…G-O-D!
PLEASE LET THIS SEAT EAT ME!

I shrank purple-faced into the purple leather seat-pad like *that* would camouflage me. "Caroline's blushing," ribbed Dad. "So, are you, sunshine?"

One of Mom's manifold pet peeves was us speaking with our mouths full. Under normal circumstances I'd gab throughout dinner expressly to display my gob's masticated contents, but *this* wasn't normal circumstances. Adhering to her table etiquette for once, stuffing in an entire roast potato and chomping tight-lipped, racking my woolly brain which 'phone call Aidan could've earwigged because I knew I hadn't confided in him, Dad repeatedly pushed, "Are you gay?" Eventually, he changed tack. "C'mon Caroline, we won't mind."

I looked at Aidan; he mouthed *Go on, they're cool.*
Nodding, I hoped that would be an end to it.
But it wasn't…

"So how long have you fancied boys then?" probed Dad.
What the fu – he's never shown any interest in me, and now he's asking…what am I supposed to say? Since Alex showed me his cock at Infants'? Fuck this! I don't need it! I need vodka an' a fag…

"SIT DOWN! WE'RE GOING TO GET TO THE BOTTOM OF THIS! I WANT TO KNOW *WHAT THE HELL* YOU'VE DONE TO KNOW YOU'RE GAY! YOU'RE FIFTEEN, FOR PETE'S SAKE! IT'S ILLEGAL 'TIL YOU'RE TWENTY-ONE!" ranted Mom, hell-bent on ruining a calm coming-out.

I looked at Aidan; he mouthed *Soz*.

"WE'LL SIT HERE ALL BLOODY NIGHT IF WE HAVE TO! *I WANT TO KNOW HOW THE HELL A SON OF MINE IS GAY!* COME ON, BIGMOUTH, I WANT ANSWERS!"

"Well, letting me wear your wedding dress and buying me dolls probably had something to do with it… And I've always liked Donna Summer and you didn't try an' stop me listening to her, did you?"

"WHAT THE HELL HAS *SHE* GOT TO DO WITH IT?!"

"Didn't you read in Nan's *Sun*? This scientist played Donna Summer to one group of mice and Beethoven to another group and the ones who listened to Donna Summer turned gay. So it's *her* fault I'm gay. Or *yours*," I accused, pouting my 'Iron Lady' lips, my white brows arched imperiously.

"YOU THINK YOU'RE SO DAMNED CLEVER, DON'T YOU? BEDROOM, NOW! DO YOUR BLOODY HOMEWORK!"

I ran upstairs, cued up a tune explicitly selected to ram my gayness down her throat, and sang along out, loud and proud,

> '*Aaaaah-I love to love you baby,*
> *aaaaah-I love to love you baby,*
> *aaaaah-I love to love you baby,*
> *aaaaah-I love to love you baby…*'

"AND YOU CAN TURN *HER* OFF OR I'LL TAKE YOUR STEREO *AND* GROUND YOU *AND* TAKE YOUR MAKE-UP *AND* STOP YOUR ALLOWANCE!"

109

I pulled the plug on Donna mid-orgasm, lay on my bed and pondered *How the fuck will she react when I get a boyfriend? I really, really, want a boyfriend...dunno where I'll find one though. Not in gay places, that's for sure...*

The closest I'd come to even a bunk-up in a gay pub had been a pie-eyed dyke I almost mistook for *Brookie*'s Terry Sullivan, whose icebreaker had been *I'm Bernard, I'm on bail for joyridin' a coach foive times over the limit.* Bernard wouldn't have it I was male. The point of *why* I'd insisted she paw my chest had been wasted when she said *Dow myther me if your tits am small*, and even after I'd made her grope beneath my tutu she'd still tried it on, propositioning, *I dow loike lickin' muff anyroad an' yow 'aven't gotta lick moyne, an' I can bum yow wi' me strap-on.*

"Listen, it mightn't bother you if the birds you fuck are men but – call me old-fashioned – the men I sleep with have to have real cocks," I'd rejected her point-blank.

And the places I like going, all the blokes I fancy are...well, fuck knows what Mark is but he isn't boyfriend material, 'cause if he is gay he isn't out, and I don't wanna have to sneak around in secret... Everyone I fancy's straight except Gay John and he's way out of my league. Why are there no gays I fancy? It's not like I'm picky or anything... But he's gotta be six foot...

Four inches taller than me, the right height difference to drape a protective arm around me, but not an eighth of an inch more or we'd be a laughing-stock.

He's gotta be thin but not skinny, and he's gotta have black hair, dyed not natural.

Because if his hair was naturally black I'd be bitter he didn't have to endure the same tiresome PMT – Prerequisite Monthly Touch-up-of-roots – as me.

He's gotta wear make-up: half the amount I do and perfectly applied. Not better applied than mine though or I'll be jealous of that as well… And he's gotta have great skin too.

Although the odd spot would be a must so I wouldn't feel like an ugly-head when I got one.

And he's gotta be amazing at givin' blowjobs and wanna give them all the time…

No, besides that I really wasn't that fussy. Mr Right had to be out there somewhere. Maybe he'd be at the Siouxsie concert next week…

8

'Love in a void...'

Siouxsie and the Banshees

We'd decamped to a dream palace, a shrine to festoon pelmets, *Lladro* and *Ligne Roset* with acres of extra footage in which to gaily steer clear of Mom. Set on a rural cul-de-sac of nine executive Tudorbethan new-builds, when our paths did cross — and with Aidan mostly out and Dad wedded to work seventy hours a week it meant *I* bore the brunt of Mom's momness — the Shires air carried our rows to our hoity-toity neighbours.

They must have pitied poor Mrs Stanley at no.2 for having to tolerate a transvestite sodomite for a son.

She's always so well turned-out too. And what she's done with her creepers on the portico trellis, it's like they've been there years. And such tasteful décor too, it's small wonder she's at her wit's end, they tsk-tsk'd.

It was a wonder the priest at no.6 and the GP at no.8 didn't pop over to propose exorcism and electric shock therapy to treat her bad seed spawn. But once they'd seen her dirty her leaded windows with 'Vote Labour' posters in the lead-up to the local election, it all became crystalline:

No wonder he's turned out the way he has. She's a hypocrite loony leftie who's benefited from wonderful Mrs Thatcher. And to think, we bought here to avoid such undesirables, they huffed.

I'd always make goddamn sure there was no avoiding me by dallying on our driveway on my way to or from town, and – when they pretended not to gawp – by appropriating an old one-liner of Boy George's which Mad Sarah had told me he fired at their nosy neighbours when she'd squatted with him during his Midlands stint:

Don't take offence dear, take the whole street!

So, the Monday of the Banshees' gig, I'd wagged school mid-morning and hurried home to get ready. Beauty-wise, I'd gone for samurai pinks and *'Aladdin Sane'* no-brows; I'd skewered my blossom-strewn coif with nacre chopsticks to compliment the dove-grey kimono I'd fashioned for the event; about to leave, I'd unhung the enormous fan from my wall – a final flourish to my *Hong Kong Garden*-inspired oriental theme which would also cool any make-up meltdowns this uncommonly torrid June; I'd railed at the snooty cow from no.7; and, desperately seeking Siouxsie – who I'd heard through the Goth grapevine would be at *The Odeon* this afternoon doing a soundcheck – I'd arrived to see there was an ocean already there. The girls, without exception, were togged up to look like their heroine. Two thirds of the geezers were as well, the remainder Sid Vicious-wannadies still safety-pinned to 1976.

Cider and spliffs did the rounds, with periodic sing-a-longs should an unfamiliar drub of a Banshees' rehearsal ad-lib familiarize itself, and morale was high until a '76 contingent of up-from-the-smoke insurgents – a fact borne-out by their Bow Bells vowels and the fact that indigenous factions coexisted peacefully – clouded the mood, angling for a fight, sneering "GOFF SHITSTABBERS!"

As they set on one Goth, the quick-thinkers among us secreted ourselves in an alcove behind the bins as the local class of '76 set on the troublemakers…bottles flying, the crunch of glass, blood-curdled cries…sirens shrieking to the scene, emergency vehicles blockading exodus from the blind-alley…truncheon-happy hooligans teeming down and forcing the unwounded into paddy wagons, paramedics hustling casualties onto ambulances…the stage-door rattling in the mayhem…as emergency services sped away, the swarm rushing forth, manners and friendships forgotten in the crush. It was everyman for himself…

Launching myself into the scrum, my cumbersome fan coming in handy to thwack opponents' shins, I elbowed all opposition aside 'til I hit a bulwark: XXXL bodyguards, walled around their charges, intent on bundling them to their Mercedes. But volatile atmospheres didn't perturb The Banshees. All-smiles, they disregarded their minders to mingle with us and scrawl the autographs we'd risked lives and limbs for, remembering they'd been us once upon a teenage wildlife, perhaps hung 'round stage-doors for the signatures of their idols: Bowie, Bolan and Brian Ferry.

With nothing for Siouxsie to sign, I proffered her my sleeve. She wrested a fabric-friendly felt-tip from someone's clutches, asked "Who to, dear?" and scribbled

To Stan, love Siouxsie Sioux.

I beat a retreat with my fan to a quiet corner, where I gazed awhile at what had transformed common cloth into a relic as sacrosanct as the Turin Shroud. Then I rifled through my bag for compact and lipgloss to attend to the secular…

"Sorry to interrupt but…"

O-H…M-Y…G-O-D!

"I just wanted to tell you I think you're beautiful."

He… he… he…

"Sorry, I'm Simon."

Six foot tall, thin but not skinny, dyed black hair and perfect make-up but not more perfect than mine, if he was amazing at blowjobs too – and with his fleshy lips, he looked like he was – Simon possessed the exact stats I'd unfussily carved in stone.

"Are you gonna tell me your name?"

"What? Sorry…I was miles away! Carl, but everyone calls me Stan."

"I'll call you Carl then. C'mon, come an' meet my friends Sandra an' Paul."

Presentations done, praise for Sandra's self-sewn stitch-for-stitch facsimile of Siouxsie's *Swimming Horses* video costume duly given, and autographs compared, the four of us ambled away. We hadn't discussed where to, but we instinctively homed in on Oasis and did a circuit, then moseyed to Rackhams' café. I was quieter than usual, combing their chatter for clues re his availability – envious of anybody they mentioned who might be his partner; not envious of asexual Paul because I intuitively knew he wasn't; but wary of Sandra because, bent as Simon may seem, they were very touchy-feely, the two of them exchanging hand-cloaked confidentialities.

"You always this quiet?" asked Paul.

"What? Oh, sorry, I was just thinking…erm…shall we go for a proper drink?"

The first pub we passed had an olde worlde sign assuring *'A Warm Friendly Welcome'* so in we went. The barman's "Ice?"

to our request for four vodka oranges was a more pertinent description of our welcome: saucer-eyed narrow minds searing with revulsion. Our unease brewing as we awaited our drinks, the barman smashed them down and snatched my fiver, then chucked my change in inconvenient coppers on the bar as opposed to in my palm.

"FUCK OFF AN' DIE, YOU FUCKIN' AIDS PUFFS," grunted a greasy bruiser.

I congratulated her on being the first pot-bellied pig I'd ever met that could walk on two legs and talk, and on being the first creature I'd encountered to use AIDS as an adjective. As I sidestepped her swinging fist, she lost her footing and crashed like a felled oak. Wasting good vodka we took flight, pounding pavements till our lungs couldn't carry us anymore…

"You're hilarious, Carl!" snorted Simon breathlessly.

"Yeah, what isn't hilarious is she must have thought I'm a tranny," Sandra tripped over her lip, femininity slighted.

"No, you're Sandrasaurus," ragged Simon.

She socked him and whinnied, "You're one puff *I* wish would fuck off an' die," which bolstered my hopes that if Simon *was* available then he might be *the one*. As Paul explained Sandrasaurus had got her nickname on account of her brontosaurus neck, Simon had an idea.

"Let's go to The Vic," he suggested.

"Only as long as Sandrasaurus winds her *looooong* homophobic neck in an' doesn't get us hetero-bashed," I said.

"I can see why Simon's got the hots for you; you're a bitchy queen too," said Sandra.

My heartstrings swirled to symphonic euphoria.

Over drinks at The Vic – a spit-and-sawdust refuge for Birmingham's dregs; its clientele rent boys and low-lives in high-heels and a hoary slipper-shod tranny with five o'clock shadow and his wig in curlers; and a continual influx of oversexed cruisers lured in by its proximity to the city's foremost cottage, the infamous Silver Slipper – and all the way back to The Odeon, Simon and I talked tonight's-probable-set-list-and-anything-but-us as Sandra and Paul only talked us-and-when's-the-wedding. But inside the auditorium our talk united to the tactics we'd use to penetrate the mosh-pit stage-front.

Interlocking arms we steamrolled in, trampling roughshod over bodies, ducking phlegm, threats fought with threats, swearing our way to within arms' reach of the footlights… joining with four thousand others' vociferous feet, slow-stamp-chanting

SIOUX-SIE, SIOUX-SIE, SIOUX-SIE, SIOUX-SIE

…her ovation as she meandered through snowflake projections crooning in an Ella Fitzgerald timbre to lullaby violins rapidly subsiding to a reverential hush…an eruption as a blinding thunderbolt struck and the pace upped to rampant Punk, the audience one pogo-ing tide, The Banshees thrashing away as tight as Siouxsie's magnesium catsuit, Siouxsie matching their every lick with energetic limb-flicks and vocal high-kicks…

Simon had slipped his hand in mine so clapping was a no-no; then, when I heckled "HONG KONG GARDEN!" for the *nth* time and Siouxsie snarled, "Fuck off and get your night bus home," he draped a protective arm around my shoulder – Siouxsie, in full-on-bitch persona, withering, "Here's something *not* from the Dark Ages 'specially for you, you loser!"

"Oh wow, fuckin' awesome! This is my favourite track off the new album," I squeaked.

"Mine too," said Simon, then plundered the deepest kiss as Siouxsie serenaded

'You're mine, you're mine all mine'

…me adoring it but anticipating I'd have to eject his tongue any minute to belt out the chorus…when he pulled away to roar "BRING ME THE HEAD OF THE PREACHER MAN" too, staring into each other, our eyes – though glowering to convey the lyrics' bloodlust – couldn't conceal that love was budding. We pogoed and sang hand-in-hand and snogged through every instrumental improv 'til last curtain, Simon asking as we filed out, "When can I see you again?"

As we chatted on the 'phone next night, I dealt the blow that I was under house-arrest for skiving yesterday – *and* I'd had my allowance withheld for flogging my clarinet which only *now,* half a year and a complete house move on, had Mom gotten wind of – until term's end. In *six weeks*…

"Look, if you don't like me just say and I'll hang up an' rip your number up an' change mine," said Simon, playing the role of lover spurned before we were officially lovers.

"No, I do…no, don't go…*please* don't do that. *Please!*" I begged, envisaging glum hours of vodka and Marc and the Mambas lying ahead.

"I'm only winding you up! I'll call you every day and I'll write too," he vowed, ringing-off with "I love you" which made me weep and wallow in a *Smirnoff* and *Torment & Toreros* cocktail anyhow…

No-one had *ever* told me *I love you.*

9

'When the fight and the folly take you further from home...'

'When The Wild Calls' Swans way

Six weeks later, every single one of those plodding 2,245,680 seconds was behind me. My suitcase on the porch, my Mohican wrought into a Mari Wilson beehive and fittingly attired for a midday flit in a cocoon of ten metres of black net, I was glopping on a fifth layer of *Helena Rubinstein* lipgloss for the road in the hall mirror, when I felt a pang that going AWOL for three weeks – Paul's parents were on vacation, Simon was staying there, and Paul had extended the invitation to me – might distress Mom. I wandered into the kitchen.

"Mom, I'm g – "
"Shush! I'm listening to this," she cut in, making it crystal clear that anything I had to say couldn't be as crucial as what anyone on *Radio 4* did...

I turned and left.

Janet called after him "F.F.Y!" her-speak to tell the kids they'd have to fend for themselves and cook their own teas tonight, but the bolshie so-and-so had already done a romper-stomper, slamming the front door so hard its panes rattled.

"DON'T DO THAT!" she hollered to nobody, switching off the radio to sample how blissful the silence would be when he'd have flown the nest forever.

The ghostly hush wasn't nice. Turning the radio on again, re-tuning to *Radio 2* in time to catch a near-hit of Marianne Faithfull's from '79 that she'd adored back then – Janet had identified with Lucy Jordan, she'd been thirty-seven too, she'd realised she'd probably never ride through Paris in a sports car with the warm wind in her hair either. Now, she was forty-two and *still* Lucy Jordan, resigned to the inevitability that, like Lucy, *she'd* go mad by the final verse of her life as well. *Well, I can't fly to Paris…I'll go up Solihull and buy an outfit with a Parisian twist, sit in that patisserie on the High Street with a pain-au-chocolat an' a café-au-lait and read my Simone de Beauvoir.*

She got herself together, slamming the front door so its panes rattled once more, and sped away, remembering all those times when her intention had been to walk out and never return, wondering what would have happened if her nerve hadn't deserted her…

★★★★

Simon ate my lipstick off on the doorstep…an unyielding kiss I'd have hiked deserts and mountains backwards-on-hands for…a film-star kiss that would've gone on longer than *Gone with the Wind* had Paul not prised us apart, light-heartedly scolding, "You two'll give that old bat across the way a coronary!"

Simon cracked open the posh fizz he'd splashed out on to commemorate our reunion, we cosied ourselves in the lounge, we exhaustively dissected Marc Almond's debut solo 45, *'The Boy Who Came Back'*, then I got all queer activist, denigrating

120

our make-up-wearing heroes for not being 'out' when it would make our lives far easier if they were.

"Jimmy Somerville's out," said Paul.

"Yeah, but *that* doesn't help us," I argued. "He doesn't even wear mascara…and he really should with those albino eyelashes… My point is, Marc, Boy George and Pete Burns are so popular that even if one of them came out and said *'I wear make-up and I'm gay but I don't have AIDS'*, we wouldn't have been called AIDS puffs just for dressing how we do."

"Carl's right," agreed Simon. "'Cause if Elton John or Freddie Mercury came out – "

"They aren't gay, are they?" I queried.

"Gayer than Larry Grayson!" laughed Paul.

"But Elton John's married. And Freddie Mercury…well, my mom loves him and she *hates* gays."

"*Pete Burns* is married, Carl. And *where* d'you think the name 'Queen' comes from?" asked Simon. "And there're rumours George Michael's gay too. He should wear a *'choose cock'* t-shirt, not *'choose life'*! But, as I was saying, you're right Carl: if Pete or Boy George or Marc came out it would help us more than Jimmy Somerville has, or if Elton or Freddie did."

That subject done, we went on to exhaustively cover other ordeals – them talking about the exams that had hampered their social lives, and me about unloving homophobe Hitler Mom who'd hijacked mine and made no secret of the fact she couldn't wait to wipe me from her life like an overdue abortion.

"You poor thing," comforted Simon.

"Simon's bricking himself about meeting her. He said she's a bit snappy whenever he 'phones yours," said Paul, topping up my champagne to help me wipe her from my life.

"Don't worry; you won't... Anyway, I haven't come here to talk about her. When are we gonna do it?" I asked, steering Simon's hand to my crotch-swell to try and turn consolation into something carnal.

"Go on, you're in my room," said Paul with no intonation we'd be abusing his hospitality if we did, and we didn't need telling twice...

Simon showed me the joys of love-making on midnight silk sheets, selfless and languid, a world away from Seb's disinterest or a mad-thrash in a Metro...from sunset to cockcrow we made love, sleepiness weighing heavy, our bodies soldered like Siamese twins, pillow-talk troths of *2gether4ever* surrendering to dreams...my reveries graciously disturbed, split-second bewilderment as my reborn peepers processed foreign surroundings, succumbing straightaway to the dreamy reality of being orally revived, Simon coaxing a twelfth blast of DNA in as many hours, then surfacing from under the covers and smacking his chops...

★★★★

Janet hadn't heard Carl come in last night. She shouted to ask whether he was coming to Winnie's. Forty minutes trapped in the car with him was rarely a joyride – they were usually at war before she'd got into second gear – but she had to admit, for all the headaches he'd caused her, heinous as he'd become, he loved his Nan and was always courteous to her. But half an hour later she'd shouted herself hoarse trying to rally the ignorant sloth, so she went alone...

"How're the boys? How's John? How's the new house?" asked Winnie.

"Great, they're doing really well, John's great, everything's great," Janet airbrushed over Aidan's anticipated A-level fails and Carl's shenanigans and the antiseptic dream home that hadn't made her marriage any more rewarding.

"Is our Carl courting?" asked Winnie.
"No, he hasn't met the right girl yet…"

She hated hearing herself play the Pollyanna, especially as that was what bugged her most about her friends who glossed over *their* delinquent sons' failings. But Winnie wasn't one for truths and if Janet started telling her the truth now, where would it end? She'd have to dig up how Winnie had henpecked Billy to an early grave; Winnie's petty resentment towards Kev's girlfriend Chris whose only misdemeanour – after she'd devotedly nursed him to his dying day – had been to wear grey to his funeral; Winnie looking down on everybody like she was some dowager duchess, which had always nettled Janet… All of that would be lost on Winnie who was chasing a chocolate éclair with a custard slice, busily living her own lie, "I dunno why I can't lose weight, Jan, 'cause I hardly eat a thing; it was carrying you for nine months made me fat, you were a huge baby."

Kev's plaque-mounted helmet insignia had pride of place on Winnie's mantelpiece, and it stoked something maternal in Janet. She couldn't conceive of losing Aidan or Carl. Would civilisation collapse if Aidan didn't get his grades and had to start uni next year? As for Carl… well, there were worse crimes than being gay, and plenty of teen offenders didn't finish up in prison. Look at Kev. He'd gone from being a pothead who'd nick from Winnie's purse to joining the force, and judging from the five-star send-off his superiors had accorded him, he'd be Chief Superintendent by now if he hadn't died…

123

When she got home, Janet peeped in Aidan's room, his desk still fatigued with books and folders from months of revision, then peeped in Carl's pigsty. *Hang on, where's his make-up?* She saw his wardrobe doors were wide open, hangers empty save his school uniform. She checked the spare room wardrobe. A suitcase had gone. She rang John at work.

"WHAT DO YOU MEAN, *DON'T FRET, HE OFTEN STAYS OUT*? FINE FATHER YOU ARE! DIDN'T YOU HEAR? HE'S TAKEN ALL HIS CLOTHES! HE COULD BE DEAD IN A DITCH!"

She hung up and hastened to Carl's room, sweeping his shelves and drawers for an address book, a diary, shuffling his things hither-and-thither but uncovering no clue, feeling under his mattress with some trepidation because once, doing the spring cleaning, she'd turned it and had unearthed a dog-eared pin-up of a buck-naked man. That had been a shocker – Carl must've only been eleven! She'd already known he did what overactive testosterone made boys do – too long in the bathroom, stained sheets sometimes – but over *men*?! She'd told herself *It's a phase* and she hadn't been under there since. *I still hope it is a phase… 'Cause what possible happiness can come from being gay? Homophobic attacks, AIDS, if he doesn't get AIDS then growing old alone? That's why I took it so badly, except I came across as angry, not concerned…*

There was nothing under his mattress, his bed neither. She searched his records, recognising some of Kev's in there; then she sat on his unmade pit, eyeing the multiple Siouxsies and Marcs eyeing her menacingly from the walls, realising she knew little about her son other than that he was crazy for them, that she didn't know his friends or where they lived, promising she'd make a concerted effort to involve herself in

124

his welfare in future and wondering how long she should wait to 'phone the police.

I'll make his bed first, perhaps read if I can concentrate, pop 'round to Maz's if I can't.

Then, something half-hidden behind his hi-fi winked at her. It was a letter.

Dear Carl, I'm so happy we met…da-de-da…falling in love… da-de-da…aah, he's got a boyfriend! She skipped to the end to identify the mystery letter writer, and then went back to where she'd got and read on. *Da-de-da-de-da-de-da…can't wait to taste your spunk…*

EUGH! I'm no prude but that turns my stomach… GOD, THIS SIMON COULD BE A PAEDOPHILE!

No, paedophiles wouldn't sign their names in heart-shape frames of kisses. He might be a psychotic murderer like Dennis Nielsen. No, murderers wouldn't sign their names like that either. There was no 'phone number, just an address, and directory enquiries couldn't help her without a surname. Now what? Drive there? Bloxwich must be over twenty miles, and at rush hour… *There's no guarantee he'll even be there… And if he is there, he'll accuse me of interfering an' it'll descend into a slanging match…*

★★★★

We watched Soft Cell's *'Non-Stop Exotic Video Show'*, which was a first for me as Mom didn't *believe* in video recorders and had vetoed Dad buying one. Afterwards, Simon suggested we call in on their friend Jabba Janis.

"She thinks she's a Goth cuz she dyes her *riah* black and wears black and all her dad says to her is 'bloody Goth'. I reckon he means G.O.T.H, as in *get out the house*," said Paul.

"She's agoraphobic," Simon chimed in.

"Her dad sounds like my mom. She's got a whole language like that so she doesn't have to waste words on me…"

Mr Janis – who resembled Sid Little – marshalled us in, fitting half a dozen audible effs into what sounded like *'Get in before the neighbours see.'* Janis, who looked like a bewigged Eddie Large – and it was on my mind to inquire, *'Who does your mom look like, Dick Emery?'* only Simon'd briefed me *Don't mention the 'm' word 'cause Janis hasn't got one* – had been keeping schtum at the furthermost end of the hallway. The second the latch clacked she lit up though, giddy to hear all our goss then not letting us get a word in edgeways, babbling nineteen to the dozen whilst uncorking the *Blue Nun* we'd brought. Considering she seldom ventured out, Janis had a cosmic knowledge of the outer world, garnered I guess from visitors and the towers of culture-bible monthlies chronologically arranged in true OCD style, and I was enjoying as fab a time as anybody could in a drab Black Country prefab bungalow when Mr Janis put a dampener on it.

"Police're here after Carl Stanley. Is that you?"

"Yes, he's Carl," Janis answered on my behalf, asking me "What've you done? Is it really bad?" then asking Simon and Paul "What's he done? Is it really bad?" fidgeting like she was about to pee, fit to burst at the prospect of being eyewitness to tomorrow's *Bloxwich Telegraph* front page. Paul shrugged.

"Whatever he's done'll be bloody disgraceful. Bloody puffs, bringin' shame on this bloody house, hurry up an' get rid of them," said Mr Janis.

"You're naughty," grinned Simon. "You never told your mom you were leaving, did you?"

The blue light, still flaring panic stations, had drawn everyone out of the neighbouring prefabs to watch.

Crockett and Tubbs conferred.

"This is definitely him, isn't it?"

"There can't be two Carl Stanleys like that."

Crockett double-checked. "For the record, you are Carl Stanley, aren't you?"

I nodded. As Tubbs paced the footpath booming numerical-code jargon into his walkie-talkie, Crockett filled me in. "A Mrs Stanley rang Solihull Police Station to report her son missing and described him as..." – he referred to his notebook – "*five-sixish, six-sixish with bouffant... thin... thick eye make-up....red lipstick... three-inch diamanté earrings...* When that was radioed through we thought it's gotta be a hoax...we get a lot of crank callers!"

Tubbs had cut the flashlight, told the crowd, "MOVE ON, THERE'S NOTHING TO SEE!" but now that they'd seen me they had judged otherwise and weren't for budging, and he'd come back to inform Crockett, "I've given the address to HQ. Mrs Stanley's on her way."

"She's comin' here? No! Why? Now you know I'm alright – "

"The law says that as you're a minor – "

"I *know* what the law says from when I was done for shoplifting! Can't you bend it just this once, *purl-e-e-e-ease*, I'm begging you! She's off her rocker...she's always taking my make-up off me, and she went mental when my brother told her I'm gay...*and* she'd go out and leave us without babysitters...*and* she walked out on my dad without us I dunno how many times... *and* she used to cane us...*and* she chucks plates at Dad! Please, please, please don't let her come an' take me! She'll convince you she's sane but I swear on Marc Almond's life she isn't! Haven't any of you seen that film *Frances*?"

"I haven't. Have you?" Crockett asked Tubbs. He shook his head. Simon, Paul and Janis – she'd overcome her agoraphobia to star in the melodrama which was making her prefab the epicentre of Bloxwich, and was galloping to-and-fro to transmit each titbit to her neighbours, risking cardiac arrest at worst, or dropping several dress sizes at best – shook theirs.

"She was this 1930s actress, she was an atheist and a communist and an alcoholic…she wasn't loopy but her mother who's a control freak was…so when she…that's Frances…assaults a hairdresser on a film set and gets fired, her mom…I can't remember who plays *her* but Jessica Lange plays Frances…persuades the doctors to lock Frances in a nuthouse which *does* send her loopy…"

From the way Crockett and Tubbs were staring at me, it was clear they thought I ought to be carted off to the nearest funny farm too.

"Christ, don't you get it? Her mom's the nutcase and so's mine! She drinks pints of gin every night and she doesn't believe in God and she's *really* left-wing… She even talks about getting rid of the royal family! Simon, if you *really* love me, *tell* them what she's like!"

Simon corroborated that, having spoken to her on the 'phone, she was everything I'd said; Paul vouched that, having known Simon for years, Simon's judgement had always been spot-on; and Janis nodded, wheezing, "Whatever they say's true!" But a cross-dressing shoplifter's character assassination and the tenuous substantiation of two fairies and an obese tittle-tattle weren't going to waive laws. Crockett said, "That's as maybe, but as you're a minor – "

"You're a fucking jobsworth! I'll give you fucking *minor!*"

I flounced indoors and resurfaced fag-in-mouth and wine-in-hand to flout two laws...extolling the delights of buggery to violate another...French kissing Simon then lighting another cig...to further grind their Pig snouts in it, quoting Quentin Crisp

> *'However low a man sinks he never reaches*
> *the level of the police...'*

Paul tagging *that* with a string of Crisp pearls which led to a four-strong sing-song of Gina X's paean to Quentin Crisp, the club-hit *'No GDM'*, with extra emphasis on the "LES-BEEE-AN" and "QUEE-AR"...me chain-smoking, the four of us carrying-on so carefree we'd forgot...

"Hello sunshine!"

I lobbed my just-lit fag.

"Hello everybody, I'm Janet," she chirruped in her finest telephone accent, sunnier than Doris Day "And this handsome chap must be..."

My jaw dropped.

What's her fucking game? Paul isn't handsome...

"I'm pleased to meet you, Paul. And you're..."

"Janis," said Fat Janis, knees buckling in a semi-curtsey.

"It's lovely to meet you, Janis. And you must be Simon! It's so nice to put a face to your voice! I bet you didn't imagine he'd have such a pleasant mother, did you? Pity he's not a chip off the old block, isn't it? He can be moody, can't he? Imagine how it is for me and Mr Stanley, we have to live with him all the time! I wish they'd hurry up and legalize gay marriage so you can take him off my hands!"

This amiable humanitarian wasn't the Mom I knew, or the ogre they'd feared. I watched them in horror, knowing they should be institutionalised for falling for her charade, copping Crockett and Tubbs shooting daggers at me, and interpreting that as *You're barmy, not her,* certain they were being conned too. Tubbs seemed so in awe of her that persons not present, shown a snapshot of his expression, would swear it was Princess Di on walkabout he was in thrall to. But Crockett hadn't forgotten why he was there.

"Mrs Stanley, what do you want to do with regards to Carl?"

"Oh, now I know he's okay he can stay here, it'll be a holiday for me! Right, sunshine, give your loving mommy a hug," she clucked, and clamped me to her breast. My blood turned to ice. She didn't do hugs, ever…

She released me and away she went – to Hell if there were any justice in the world – then off zoomed the officers to someplace they might actually be useful. The neighbours slithered away – no doubt pondering what this embodiment of Saint Anne had done to beget an amoral devil of a son like me – and then there were five. Mr Janis padded-out what sounded like *'They should've taken you an' locked you up an' thrown away the key'* with fourscore perceptible effs; and Simon, Paul and Janis all gushed how fortunate was I having a mom *sooo* cool, *sooo* nice, Mom this, Mom that, eulogising her TV ad just-stepped-out-of-a-salon halo and *Jaeger* cruisewear like they were saintly attributes. And I could almost pardon motherless Janis for going gaga over Mom, but not Paul whose mom – from what he'd said – really was cool and nice, and definitely not mommy's boy Simon who was meant to adore only *me*!

Even after we'd left Janis's and were back at Paul's, his and

Simon's Mom-fest continued...on and on...*Shut up!* ...and on...*SHUT THE FUCK UP!*...and on and on...

"I'm going upstairs," I said, and galumphed up to trawl Paul's records for an accusatory tune to blare out and test Simon's love, settling on The Human League's nine-minute minimalist remake of *'You've Lost That Loving Feeling'*, its protracted intro affording me a full three minutes to assume an aptly forsaken foetal pose upon the bed for him to find me in when he came running...

By verse two he had...

"Carl, what's wrong?" he petitioned again.
Still I didn't reply, pressing my victor's grin into the bedding...
"Are you crying?"
...gnashing my molars and gnawing my lower lip...
"What is it, Carl?"
...grunting through my nose...
"Do you think I've lost that loving feeling?"
...my body a tremor, eyes watering from straining to suppress treacherous giggles.

Simon lay behind me and moulded his body to mine, murmuring "Because I love you more than anyone or anything," re-avowing his love again, and that he'd sooner die than upset me. Somewhere along the line truth triumphed over treachery and triggered a teardrop...life's lows leaking in and spawning another tear and another and another...tears soon untamed, snot bubbling, blubbing "It's not you, it's me" as Phil Oakey, well into the subsequent track by now, droned

'of youth and other madness'

131

Simon sprang up, turned Phil off and fetched tissues, urging me – before I suffocated from crying - to sit up. I did.

"Do you want to talk about it, Carl?"

I shook my head, picturing myself an un-fanciable semolina-faced wreck, afraid to look at him, my gaze moored on my splodgy Boots *No. 7* imprinted on the pillowcase like inkblot psychiatry till what I saw – Mom's mascara cesspools after every time she tested Dad – frightened me too. Punching it, punching *her*, welling up afresh from the fear that *her* ills might've infected me, I shoved it to the floor.

"Carl, what is it? What can I do to cheer you up?"

"You can suck me off," I sniffled, too wearied even to think of more weeping, banking on an Elastoplast blowjob to patch up my punctured ego *and* plug a looming waterfall that was mightier than my self-control.

Forcing my face to his, he brokered a bargain, "Only if you smile."

I feigned an Ultrabrite beam, he busied himself honouring his side of the pact with a lover's zeal, and afterwards, when he asked "Did that do the trick?" I – genuinely grinning, adding *'cure-all'* to sex's other benefits – answered

"Yeah, it did."

Lethargic weeks whizzed when all I had to do was trowel on my warpaint, scoff Paul's cooking, and lie there while Simon bestrode me or his therapeutic lips subdued my demons. But all good things come to an end...

★★★★

Janet was pottering as she waited for the milk for their bedtime Horlicks to boil. She was just about to fold up that day's *Guardian* and chuck it away when she remembered she'd not yet cut out the Philip Larkin poem they'd printed in their piece on *'Contenders for Poet Laureate'*. She Blu-tacked it at eye-level to the unit front above where she kept her handbag, where it'd be a daily reminder that *her* faults were Winnie's and Billy's, that as a mother – *and father* she groused, cramming the newspaper into the Brabantia which John *still* hadn't got 'round to emptying – she had only ever tried her best, that she must've done something right because her kids, while they might not be paragons of virtue, weren't heir to her depressive traits…

★★★★

As I trekked the last mile from the night bus terminus to home-sour-home, hatred toward Mom for that debacle at Janis's bred the nearer I got. The scab of twenty nights ago, that painful insight I'd had at Paul's that *I* was like *her*, was itching. The lights were off. Figuring I was due damages for what she had done to me, freezing two ticks to gauge whether my suitcase had woken her or Dad when I'd dropped it letting myself in, about to dip into her handbag I saw a cutting on the cupboard door:

> *'They fuck you up, your mom and dad.*
> *They may not mean to but they do.*
> *They fill you with the faults they had*
> *And add some extra, just for you.'*

Is she having a fuckin' laugh?!
In her handbag was a richly-stuffed envelope; she'd been to the bank today.
Fuck nicking a fiver! Her filling me with all her shit an' sticking that up there…that's gotta be worth way more than a fiver…

133

A trillion Krugerrand wouldn't have compensated, but I wasn't avaricious. I restricted myself to a pound for each dolorous year I had been alive. Plus another five for any future agonies her genes might inflict on me...

Twenty quid would do...for now.

10

'Playing with fire gets you burnt...'

'Midnight' Yazoo

Simon and I hooked up every other day and dawdled around our habitual haunts, or we'd slouch beneath the sycamores of Pigeon Park where Punks and Goths would preserve their lily-white tans in the baroque shadow of St Philip's. Come dusk we'd drift to The Vic where we'd dry-hump till he had to scram for the last 51 bus to make his last connection to backwoods Bloxwich.

Frustratingly left with a woody *again*, my libido led me down the fusty steps of the Silver Slipper. It reeked of disease. At the urinals, a line of Joes – whose blatantly jerky hands categorically weren't helping them urinate straight – craned their necks in unison and stared. Even if *that* hadn't been so daunting, even if one pursed face hadn't said *You're in the wrong loo dear, this is the Gents*, I'd have been hard-pressed to stand there masturbating in an ankle-length fishtail skirt, so I hobbled to the stalls to save face and look as if I'd come to dump, killing time thinking *What're you doing here? Simon worships you.* But when an erection penetrated the partition wall glory hole, I justified *Simon never lets me suck him off* – our first night versatility having swiftly flatlined to an Arthur and Martha predictability where I was unfailingly Arthur. I stooped to pleasure it, but its Stilton stench was so unpalatable I bolted in disgust – disgusted by it, by the place, at myself for going there – declaring total chastity to Simon and only wavering once when I went clubbing, and whored myself in a car park afterwards for ten cigs and a saveloy. And in the midst of a global recession *that* didn't count...

Her poetic gibe aside, Mom'd been suspiciously cordial since I'd come back from Paul's. On one occasion she'd even been complimentary about my make-up. Mistrustful of her motives, sure I must have done a botch-job and it was some venomous ploy to send me out looking crap, I'd exhausted myself checking my reflection for flaws. Finding none, I began to dare to trust her sincerity. As soon as I did that, she went back to her old sardonic self...

"What with this house being spotless, and your track record of throwing hair dye *all over* the carpets at the old house, we've decided that – as you can't be trusted to be left alone – when we go to Aberaeron at half-term you're coming too."

Her infringement of my civil liberties put me in a matricidal temper.

"SO IT WAS ALRIGHT TO LEAVE A NINE YEAR-OLD FOR DAYS ON END BUT NOW I'M FIFTEEN AN' THREE QUARTERS IT ISN'T?"
"DROP THE ATTITUDE OR WE'LL CHANGE OUR MINDS! ZIP IT AND LET ME FINISH! We've decided you can invite Simon."

"*What?* After the palaver you made over me being gay?"
"Nonsense, you're making it up! I'm broad-minded, I always have been. I love Queen!"

136

Since I'd be abducted to Wales anyway, and my inflexible spine prohibited auto-fellatio, and dead-hand soap-wanks were no substitute for Simon's orifices, sexual frustration decreed I agree...

Competitive Dad was in his Nigel Mansell bubble, ignoring the speed limit, determined to overtake every motorist; Mom and Simon were nattering like bosom buddies and getting along too well for my liking; and I, huffily silent, dug his thigh now-and-again to remind him *I am here*. He grated on me more and more as he snickered at her reminisces:

Black-haired rat...
He used to play with dolls...
The pansy was so body-shy he wouldn't take
his vest off at the seaside...

Simon remained impervious to my hints until my huffs, elongated and louder with Mom's every humourless embarrassment, silenced him. He squeezed my knee as Mom performed to an audience of one – herself – and I shunned him for a few junctions. When I deigned to look his way, he pouted penitently. I gave him an *I-forgive-you* peck. I was gagging that badly for a shag and a fag – and to get away from *her* – that Dad couldn't make the impressionistic vistas siding the A5 fly past fast enough...

Mom eschewed her women-are-the-stronger-sex ideologies to issue the order "You men can unload the car!" then swanned in to recce the Regency terrace. She allocated Simon and I the rear gable room – gesturing at my ghetto-blaster, explaining "Your din shouldn't spoil our holiday from up there...now go an' unpack and keep out of our way 'til dinnertime."

The instant we entered our room I ferreted in my holdall for my poppers and the specially compiled mix-tape I'd initialled 'S' for 'sex', whisked my kit off, and swooped so rashly on Simon – folding and hanging his apparel, diligent as a *Benetton* shopgirl – that the seagrass flooring burnt my kneecaps. To a debauched soundtrack which included Velvet Underground's *'Venus in Furs'*, I actively reversed our butch-and-bitch roles for the duration of Side A before flipping both it and Simon over for the duration of Side B. That honeymoon thrill had been recaptured – I couldn't have fancied any man more. If Matthew Ashman had abseiled in starkers bearing a stiffy more impressive than Wolverhampton Mark's, with all the vodka in Russia and all the marijuana in Morocco I might have even rebuffed *him*…

The whole restaurant lapped us up. Everyone bar the parochial waitress ushering us to our seats – who was too taken in by the good-looking gentleman's *thank-you-my-love-how-are-you-my-love* routine to notice the outlandish teenagers and glamorous head-turner in tow – the waitress twinkling brighter when Dad, without checking prices, ordered, "Two bottles of your finest red, my love." Peeved, Janet's disgruntlement didn't stem from envy; *she* wasn't jealous of some frowzy Blodwen! It was irritation; irritation that some-one else had fallen for it. But they always did. They'd never guess that Mr Flash-the-cash could be a right penny-pincher when it suited; or that Mr Charm had, unbeknownst to his wife, authorized her ECT; or that in twenty-seven years he hadn't once told her she was beautiful…

Dad was schmoozing with the party at the adjoining table. Simon, Mom and I were done assassinating those diners resistant to fashion, and conversation had veered to politics.

When I hailed the Iron Lady, Mom repented, "Shame the Brighton bomb didn't kill her!"

"Well *I* like her. She's made Britain great again," I said.

"You don't know what you're talking about! *You* don't watch the news or read a paper. She's a homophobic – "

"*You* don't know what you're talking about, *mother!* Go to a gay bar, they make *me* homophobic!"

"…megalomaniac. Dismantling the unions, privatisation, she's destroying industry bit by bit."

"Well, *Dad's* business is booming. And *you* voted for her!"

"That was the biggest mistake of my life…well, the *second* biggest," she said, tilting her head at me.

She proceeded to re-run her hackneyed *black-haired rat* repertoire which Simon – by now under the influence of two sips of Cabernet Sauvignon – found wittier than ever. Then she saw fit to dredge up my shoplifting, and add that just last Wednesday Dad had had to fit a lock on the spare bedroom where their cashbox was because she'd nabbed me red-handed, *and* that Simon would've been uninvited were they not such lenient parents. She edited out the fact that she'd gone all Muhammad Ali on me and had then browbeaten Dad till he pummelled me too.

"Anyway, that's enough about *him*, what about *you* Simon?"

He's nice enough but he's not Carl's equal, thought Janet, zoning out as Simon inflated his CSE passes as if he'd passed five degrees. *Same with Steph, she's not in Aidan's league…God, listen to yourself, you're as judgemental as Mom! I just don't want my kids to settle for less like I did.* She recalled the missed opportunities, the wrong turns… the debonair son of GKN's president wooing her…. rejecting him because she was betrothed to John… her girlhood fantasy that she'd marry

Mario Lanza and live a diamond life in his strawberry-sorbet palazzo in Palm Springs with servants and squillions of dollars… Billy counselling her at the altar *It isn't too late to change your mind, Jan*… the nagging worry that her sanity was ebbing away like a leaky water tank... She pushed her thoughts away, and re-tuned her attention to Simon…

The gigglier Mom and Simon got, the more hacked off I got, clinking my cutlery murderously. I'd have stabbed her in the fucking eyeball with my fork if I'd thought it might shut her up for one second. I had other plans for Simon. Contriving another loyalty test, at my impatient behest we left Mom and Dad to their Irish coffees to go for a stroll through the drowsy fishing village. The natives' comments – all squiggly absurdities which in all probability were Welsh for *Fuckin' AIDS puffs* – had us hoot 'til our eyeliner ran, rather than cack our pants. *Now we're on our own and everything's perfect, I'm not gonna do what I was planning*, I told myself; but down by the quay, the combination of mist and serious moonlight and indigo turbulence was too irresistibly *French Lieutenant's Woman* to resist, and – as if I had Tourette's – the words, "I think we should split up" spilt out of my mouth.

Desolation dissolved his smile…Simon blubbering "Why?…Why?…Why?"…imploring "Why say it?" when I said, "I don't mean it, I'm only playing!"…admonishing, "You can't mess with my emotions Carl!" when I began to blubber and implore his forgiveness…Simon brushing my hand away when I went to hold his, and calling my bluff, "I want to break up before you drive me insane." No amount of snivelling would sway him to reconsider, and in bed that night, when I rubbed my hard-on against him, positive that *that* would mend us, he built a pillow barricade between us. It may as well have been The Berlin Wall…

Not only did the wall stay, but for six days he wouldn't even speak. If I entered a room, he left it. In the car going on excursions, he consumed magazines he'd already worn out from cover to cover, continuously welded to his Walkman. We went to an electric cliff railway from where – allegedly – the panorama on a clement day was the most splendid in the British Isles (but the afternoon we went up was blanketed in cement-grey clouds) and he kept away from me. We visited what the guidebook said ranked amongst Europe's most glorious medieval fortresses (in fact one decayed turret trellised in scaffolding) and he avoided me. He snubbed me on days out to a honey museum, to a taxidermy museum, to Aberystwyth…which were all as sickeningly dull as they sound, and even duller with no-one to talk to.

Then, on the last night, he confessed, "I still love you," removed that pillow wall and orchestrated sex.

"That was amazing! Can we forget this week and start again?" asked Simon as I lit a post-coital *Marlboro*.

"Sorry Simon, you can't go changing your mind just 'cause we had sex; how can I be sure you won't dump me again? *You* ended it, remember," I said, laying the entire onus for our situation on him, underscoring every second word with staccato Bette Davis drags.

"Only because *you*…oh, it doesn't matter now…I'll always love you…and I *never* lost that loving feeling, not even when I saw you go down The Slipper."

"*What?* I didn't do anything!"

"Sorry Carl, we're through. Maybe we can be friends in time but it'll take me a long time to get over you," he said, his sentence punctuated with snuffles, climbing into bed and wrapping himself in eiderdown.

Extinguishing the light, climbing in and motioning to cuddle him, his muffled voice reiterated "It's over." He shifted over to the farthest perimeter. The chasm between us felt wider than the cosmos. Totting up how long it had been from love at first sight to these irreconcilable differences, grieving how in only 137 days it had come to this, when I was certain he was asleep, snoring that faint snore of his I'd never hear again, I sobbed too, agonising *Will I ever be loved again? Will I be more or less myself now I'm single?*

Depressed, I returned to school with my hair scraped flat in a ponytail and devoid of make-up. I meekly endured a myriad of "GOT AIDS YET?" – the punchline to the Thin Knots' unfunny gag "What does *gay* mean?" Every night I did my homework without Mom nagging me to, always to the gossamer strains of Cocteau Twins played at an unobtrusive volume. For two weekends – instead of painting the town – I knuckled down to revision for next month's mocks. I hadn't even had a wank…

"Simon hasn't rung lately; have you two had a tiff?" nosed Mom that Monday morning, counting out my lunch money.

"We broke up."

"Aw, that's a pity, I like Simon. He's had a lucky escape though, you aren't the easiest individual to get on with," she dispensed solace-for-the-heartbroken in her own inimitable manner. Re-reading that yellowing poem still stuck on the cupboard door, the spleen flooded in thick and fast.

Fuck her, fuck Simon, and fuck being late for school!

I stamped upstairs, blasted that *'fuck the mothers kill the others, fuck the others kill the mothers'* lambaste whilst tussling with my tail comb, and the closer my hair got to God, the more my defiance soared. *And fuck revising 'cause who needs O-levels?* There'd be no mope-in-my-room conscientious scholar this weekend or any other. Backcombed to epic proportions, my eyes profanely pencilled, with my porcelain heart bubble-wrapped and unbreakable, it would be don't-fuck-with-me from now on.

11

'And suddenly the picture was distorted....'

'Hall of Mirrors' Kraftwerk

"Where've you been: holiday or Strangeways?"

"I've been around, it's just that I had a boyfriend for four months and I only went clubbing once while we were together," fell on deaf ears.

"You've been away an *aeon* missed you enormously while you were gone you missed the inception of Gay John's latest conception you *have* to come tonight it won't be *nearly* a fraction as much fun if *you* don't come," overplayed Psycho Steve in his nonstop rhythmical rhetoric.

We'd only spoken the once. He'd blitzed me with a breathless soliloquy that time too – that time for an hour – although all I'd actually gleaned was that he'd drawn his eyebrows on in indelible marker-pen using a protractor as a template in 1982 and they'd been there ever since, and that his mentality see-sawed from euphoric to morose and back again each minute. I'd presumed this psychological imbalance was the genesis of his epithet – not his psychedelic garb or the tattered copy of Pink Floyd's LP *'The Piper at The Gates of Dawn'* which he'd been carrying then and was carrying today...

"Come to The Kipper Club please promise you'll come say 'I promise I'll come' *please*," he wept, his maroon lips aquiver, shoulders shrunk in the guise of a Pierrot.

Not wishing to tip him over the edge in Rackhams' café, I swore "I'll come, I promise!"

His frown instantly flip-flopped to a grin. Steve winded me with an overzealous bear clinch which belied his scrawniness, and – in the process – asphyxiated me with the noxious talc crust that masqueraded as his skin. Wiping his epidermis off my top, memorising his footstep-by-footstep talking-map of how to get there, I threw him off-balance anyway by declining his offer of tea so I could race home to hem an ensemble I'd been toiling over all week: a white satin dress with gold-and-white lace fins fanning from its tulip skirt side-seams, handkerchief sleeves in the same lace, and a gold lamé bodice.

I dropped by Rackhams' haberdashery department on the off-chance I'd discover something to lend it that additional *je ne sais quoi*, and nicked an ornamental white dove and a spool of white satin ribbon. Black hair, black eyeshadow and red lipstick – and the red label *Thunderbird* I'd buy to guzzle on the bus back into town – were the only colours which would deviate from my gold and white palette. And fuck the winter frost that was upon us; I'd channel Sandie Shaw and go out shoeless because no one did that.

Nimbly treading the unswept nettle-fissured backstreets of Birmingham's dilapidated factory district, and up two flights of a sinister walk-up – climbing the stairs past camel-coated Arthur Daley types guffing into mobile handsets as hefty as breeze blocks – Gay John was at the door looking hotter than July even if his Adonis physique *was* hidden beneath a baggy zoot suit.

"Hello there, stranger," said John. "You look great, barefoot an' bootiful! Stan, Nick, Nick, Stan. Don't charge Stan, he's VIP."

The deliciously impish Mohican till-boy he'd spoken to vaulted over the counter to hug me like a long-lost brother.

John escorted me in – it was very empty, I was very early – to introduce me to the barmaids, Nicole and Jennifer, both resplendent in instantly recognisable *Kahn & Bell* ruched dresses.

"Whaddya wanna drink?'" asked John.

I wanted to say *You*, but as he'd never fancy me and rejection would be too demoralising, I replied, "Double vodka and half a lager and a white wine spritzer all in a pint glass, please, with a touch of lime to take the edge off it."

"Don't charge Stan, he's one of the family," said John.

After they'd fixed my drink, Nicole and Jennifer tottered from around the bar and embraced me as enthusiastically as Nick had. We chinked glasses to toast my initiation into the clan. *This is one family I want to be part of,* I thought. *A family of choice, not accident…*

Things had really kicked-off the previous evening. Mom, peeling spuds, had muttered some snideness about my dissolute fags-and-booze-and-drugs lifestyle – she'd found my ashtray and vodka empties and poppers in my wardrobe – and blamed that as being the cause of my pimple. "Poppers aren't drugs," I corrected her, highlighting her crow's feet in retaliation. She'd sprung at me, blustering rancour and brandishing the knife, its blade swashing worryingly near to my jugular. I'd grabbed her wrist to wrest it from her when Dad appeared.

"JOHN! HELP! HE'S TRYING TO STAB ME!" she screamed.

If Aidan hadn't come in and wrestled Dad off me – he'd tackled me to the cushioned lino and I'd learned its manufacturer could've been less stingy with its cushioning properties – Dad would have committed infanticide. That hadn't been the first time Aidan had done that though, although details of that instance were sepia scintillas entombed in the '70s. Mom had truly mislaid her marbles this time. I wondered whether Mom's violent psychosis would diminish my circumstances adequately to qualify for a council flat, because – if not – who'd insure I'd see my seventeenth year once Aidan escaped her luncay to go to university September next?

Gay John gave me the lowdown on the venue. This decrepit slut of a strip joint, whose erstwhile voluptuous upholstery now sagged and where nipple tassels hadn't gyrated in generations, had been sister club to The Fantasy Club downstairs. That explained those spivs on the stairs.

"It's the ideal place for a contemporary burlesque revue, isn't it?" asked John.

Natalie Wood bump-and-grinding her assets as burlesque queen Gypsy Rose Lee was all the exposure I'd had to burlesque, and tough though it was to fathom how big bucks Hollywood could possibly transfer to this diminutive speakeasy's flaky gilt stage, assuming *contemporary* was the keyword, I readily agreed.

"Well, you'll *luuurve* it," assured John. "Soz Stan, it's getting busy, better do some hosting. Show's at 11.30, don't miss it!"

Blagging another cocktail, torn between dancing to Visage's newie, *'Love Glove'* – which had underwhelmed dancers and cleared the dancefloor to present the perfect opportunity to show-off my new gown – or salvaging my bitch-status (which must have slid since I'd been away so long),

147

I sidled across to the scene's biggest bitch, Curtain Mark, who was parading his newest-in-a-long-line-of-made-from-curtains duster coats.

"You shoulda left that on your nan's window," I said.

"Fuck off, Stan…what's that pigeon on the side of your head? And what're them rags in your hair? Least I can afford *real* extensions," he swanked, pawing his acrylic rats' tails.

"You're lucky that yak didn't kick you in the face when you plucked its fucking arse!"

"Fuck off, Stan. I'll kick *you* in the face with my gazelle-like legs if you ain't careful," warned Mark, high-kicking a knobbly fishnet leg, then stubbing out his fag on somebody's Vivienne Westwood, then shifting his venom onto Black Andrew. "Ooh look, she's got her cocoa powder out again!"

Andrew's pathological fear of sebum meant he'd spend most of his night mattifying his T-zone, and when he wasn't eroding his *Flori Roberts* compact he'd be white-lying "I'm Diana Ross's love child." He'd have us believe that – as mothering a bastard in 1968 would've exterminated her megastardom – Miss Ross had surrendered him to a family of West Indians in West Bromwich.

"If I was Diana Ross and my son had Moira Stewart's head I'd 'ave had him adopted too," crowed Mark. While Andrew blotted away, indifferent to Mark who'd broken into a chorus of *'Someday We'll Be Together'*, Tracey, a firecracker who always wore grown-up baby-grows, whose tufted bob was the colour and texture of Orville, had toddled over to impart her beauty wisdom.

"Staneth, you're only supposed to use white eyeliner on your inside rims to open up your eyes, *not* to draw eyebrows on," she said, splaying her Kewpie doll eyes as wide as they'd go to illustrate her point.

"Fuck off, Trace. What the fuck do you know? You look like you've got conjunctivitis, your eyebrows look like fucking tadpoles, and your mascara's lumpier than – "

I was about to say *Angie Watts'*, when Susie, the classiest personification of Goth, interjected, "Mad Marie just offered me 50p to watch her piss!"

"I'd watch her *shit* for 50p," said Curtain Mark.

"You'd *eat* her shit for 50p," I quipped.

"I'd pay anythin' to eat Tina Turner out," cherub-cheeked Batty Patty lowered the tone, detailing exactly how she'd do it…

Just when Patty's description of cunnilingus was becoming too gross to stomach; just when apologetic Psycho Steve ran in addressing nobody in particular *Sorry I'm late did I miss anything The Kipper Club's great* – straight past me, fortunately, and bear-hugging and asphyxiating Mad Sarah *and* Patti Bell in one fell swoop – an alarm call of *WATCH OUT! HERE I COME!* drew the whole club to the dancefloor like a magnet…bodies battling for meagre floor space…as the rhythm hit, the heavens astir with hands–in–the–air mimicking its synthesizer hand-claps, everyone spazzing out to new-out *'You Spin Me Round (Like A Record)' (Performance Mix)*…everybody except Tracey who only liked Patti LaBelle, and had only come to dance because everyone else had… Tracey swaying perfunctorily and griping noisily "I HATE THIS SHIT!" for the full seven minutes twenty seconds…

The instant Dead or Alive died away, my unshod feet grazed and singed, it was back to Jennifer and Nicole to blag a third cocktail – strictly medicinal – to anaesthetise my disco-wounds. The glamazonian Maggie De Monde, Birmingham's answer to Rita Hayworth who was one third of the band Swans Way was at the bar, and a Top Twenty hit, *'Soul Train'*, hadn't enlarged her ego and she was as tipsily chatty as ever. Then, tip-toeing a cautious trail to the Ladies, I stopped to ask a gangly giant – his physiognomy as non-figurative as a Picasso, with bogey green dreadlocks coiled in a ginormous topknot caged in chicken wire – "Why have you only got half a beard?"

His riposte was a cascade of giggle-gabble. Subtitles wouldn't have gone amiss. But amid the jabberwocky I did divine *half a razor*. I laughed. Half-a-Beard set sail on another stream of gibberish, waving his index finger, upon whose tip was a miniscule square. Nod-nod-nodding like I understood everything, even the bit involving elephants and gravy and a Rubik's cube, I was so chuffed at deciphering *Open your mouth* that I did. In shot his finger, he handed me his pint, and – much as snakebite-and-black and me disagreed – with that papery square sapping my juices and my tongue Sahara-dry, what harm could one tiny sip do? He leered devilishly and began to babble about *'it'* unlocking magical doors, I think, and trips to wonderland, I think. Intrigued though I was, I was also desperate to wee before show-time – which, as Gay John was doing the rounds to round up his cast, was imminent – so I left him jabbering amongst himselves…

To a crackly Brechtian recording, Gay John – topless, glitter-sprayed, and top-hatted – gusted through the tatty russet drapes, arms outstretched to bathe in our rapturous adulation, basking in it just long enough for him not to seem narcissistic.

"FUCK YOU! FUCK YOU ALL VERY MUCH FOR COMING ALL OVER ME!" he growled masochistically, strutting the semi-circular stage and lashing his microphone flex. "BITCHES UND GERMS…and those in between…

I AM GAY JOHN! MY DISOBEDIENT DOG-ETTES ARE FROTHING AT THE GASH TO ENTERTAIN YOU WITH DITTIES AN' TITTIES AN' GENERAL DEPRAVITY, SO, WITHOUT FURTHER ADO, FIRST OUT OF THE KENNEL, I PRESENT..." – he paused for dramatic effect – "TWIGGY!!!"

The curtains juddered apart, and Twiggy, looking like some sci-fi dominatrix, mimed *'The Twist'* – not Chubby Checker's trite original but Klaus Nomi's obscure, operatic, trippy re-imagining. On the final note, Gay John flew from the wings to lead the applause and announce the second act: sumo-sized Jah Wobble, dragged-up *à la* Widow Twanky, making Gilbert and Sullivan twirl in their graves by corrupting one of their innocent operettas with gratuitous gusset-rubbing and finger-sniffs…

Day-Glo droplets started dripping on me from above. Glancing up to determine their source I scoured…and scoured…and scoured…so absorbed in nothingness I didn't hear Gay John herald Julie…insentient that Julie was even onstage until I heard Mad Sarah jeer, "BEDWELL BY NAME, BED BAD BY NATURE!" It was an adage Sarah had coined after Julie had compelled Gay John to let her give him a blowjob. When he'd got it out Julie had blown on it, and Sarah had been shaming her about it forevermore.

Drawn back to the show, Julie – a dead ringer for Diana Dors of yore – was writhing in lingerie to a beat so dirty it should have been illegal. Despite Sarah, the straight guys were universally slobbering like dogs on heat as Julie squished her DD's, then rotated 180° so her back was to us and leant to touch her toes and wiggle her derriere which was spared from sheer indecency only by the merest wisp of G-string. Julie's lap-dogs wolf whistled wildly. Dip-wiggling again, tracing her

151

fingers in crevices where theirs longed to linger, as Julie milked them to near orgasm I saw them all bollock-naked, boners everywhere. But I couldn't trust my eyes, not when they'd misled me over those Day-Glo droplets...

Resisting the temptation to grab a cock I wasn't *even* sure was real, wanting verification this really *was* happening, passing on Mad Sarah to my left and Batty Patty in front – those prefixes weren't satirical – I turned to Janet on my right, who, despite her crazy paving teeth, Silly String hair and a forename shared with Mom, was pretty sane. By now, Julie was taking her bows, not a dry Jap's eye in the house as they showered her in appreciation. I went to speak but in a cock-eyed blink they'd all gone, not a wiener, not even a weensy limp one anywhere...

Then, uncertain whether I *did* see some Punky tranny feed her chocolate starfish a Mars Bar in entertainment's name – and unsure precisely how many artistes had disgraced the stage or how long had elapsed since the show's end... and *did* the walls ripple? Or was it an optical illusion, reflections from the mirrorball? ...and yes, my eyes told me that they *did* see vampiric The Count Porl squeeze his claret-splattered *Teeny Weeny Tiny Tears* so it puked green gunk, because that was his customary greeting, but... really? ...and, on the dancefloor frugging to The B-52s' *'Rock Lobster'*, was an added confusion....

Is the ground spinning or is it me?

I stopped dancing and when *it* didn't, I steadied myself on the handrail at the dancefloor's edge, my brain awhirl, raking the club-scape for anyone or anything static – because on top of the chaotic circulation of revellers even the fixtures and fittings were in flux. My eyes finally settled on a cardboard cut-out of Julie whose platinum mane and white cocktail frock radiated a Tinkerbell glow under the UVs. I'd barely collected my senses when Julie's likeness waved at me – an exaggerated Jayne Mansfield wave which roiled the ether to a tempestuous whitecap so perilous it would sink continents. Clenching the handrail for dear life, I tried to yell

I CAN'T SWIM!

but parting my lips felt like tearing a slice of mozzarella pizza…gulping a lungful of air just before the surf tore away the rail and imbibed me…colliding with the seabed…a survival instinct advising *Hold your breath and you'll float up…* cannoning past shoals of humanoid rainbow-parrotfish water-pedalling to an indistinguishable gurgle from sodden speakers…towards and yon the ocean's surface…up… up… up…built brick-by-brick stone-by-stone until I'd grown Empire State human, my cranium skimming the ceiling, hunch-necked…a bird's-eye view, neon dots boogieing like cells viewed through a microscope lens…down… down…. down… smaller and smaller till shoes were big as buildings… scurrying underneath stiletto-sole arches, fearful I'd get bayoneted by killer heels…small hazard of *that* happening once it dawned *I'm normal height again.*

Now I was safe, attempting to dance but moving as if I were in Araldite, at the epicentre of a kaleidoscope of gemstone snowflakes transmogrifying into ever more intricate formations all flashing Cheshire Cat smiles, one smile contorted to a scowl…the scowl belonging to a Lego nun condemning

You'll go to Hell for stickin' that kipper up my fucking snatch…

the incensed nun aiming a lipstick at me like a gun, ruby globs spewing from its barrel and mutating in space…marvelling *Wow, I'm inside a lava lamp*…a blissful sensation because…

'*Sun arise come…*' wailed Alien Sex Fiend's Nik Fiend on '*Ignore the Machine*'…

…now the music had…

'*…every-y-y-y…*'

…had gone...

'*…m-o-o-o-orning*'

…had gone gluey too, I was…

*'Br-i-i-i-inging b-a-a-a-ack the w-a-a-a-armth
to-o-o-o-o the grou-u-u-u-und'*

…I was…

Why's Dad shaking me?

…if only my thoughts would stop, I'd be almost on the beat …

AIDAN, STOP HIM! I DON'T WANNA BE HERE! I WANNA…I wanna be…I…I…

*'I live in Siberia
through no fault of my own'*

…*I wanna be back in the club, back where I…*

'A blank generation in the danger zone'

...I...I...I'm...

Different clubs, different styles of music and clothes and hair, struggling to find the beat all through the '80s and into the '90s, those same fragmented thoughts of Dad shaking me when I was a child still haunting me whenever I least expected...

...now that my Acid had kicked-in I was finally dancing in time...surrounded by legions of Golliwogs in wheelchairs that had commandeered the floor to *do-si-do*.

I danced across to a nude slave-boy on a leash who'd plied me with beers earlier then accompanied me on all fours 'til my bladder was ready to recycle it and he could drink it, and dribbled, "How did they get up the stairs?"

I didn't know what drugs he was on, but they'd numbed his ability to articulate.

The room imploding into an origami fortune teller had been adorable, but disabled Golliwogs – who were now blaming me for slavery – weren't. Trial and error had taught me that, for me, coke or valium levelled out LSD. I bent to forage in my sock. An anonymous hand, mistaking it as a come-on, kneaded my buttocks, bare in jockstrap and leather chaps. I let his digits wander, because at *Fist* – a lesbian-run monthly London fetish night held in a crumbling warehouse – being the buffet was par for the course. Here, once they'd got past its skinhead door-whore Polly who implemented *Fist*'s stringent 'fetish wear only' admittance policy with authoritarian inelasticity, man-sluts came to enact their wildest

155

fantasies and, while their rocks reloaded, to dance to nosebleed techno. I'd got the wrong sock. In this one I'd stashed my last will and testament which read:

> *If I take a bad E or OD on K and die tonight,*
> *I died having a fabulous time!*

Should drugs devour me, unscrupulous hacks weren't going to bowdlerize my demise as they had Leah Betts', and let's face it, my sordid death – by my association to the lady who until five years prior had been the western world's most powerful woman, whose sometime make-up artist I was – was bound to be newsworthy…

★★★★

"My eyesight isn't what it was but I can feel from the touch of your brush that you have given me a mouth like Brigitte Bardot. Thank you," she'd cooed the first time I'd done her.

Her vain squint – a squint which had overseen the sinking of the battleship *Belgrano*; a squint that had perused and endorsed the anti-promotion-of-homosexuality bill, Clause 28; a squint to domineer her sceptical crony ministers to levy The Poll Tax which had precipitated her eviction from Number 10 – overstrained to scrutinise my handiwork.

"No, thank *you*, Prime Minister," I said, observing yet again the protocol her office had stipulated.

"*No, no, no,* dear. I'm no longer Prime Minister. It warms me that *you* still consider me your leader but *please* call me Maggie. I like Maggie. Maggie is *so* motherly, *so* approachable. Now jot down the make and colour of this lipstick, my dear!"

As the photo-shoot drew to a close, Maggie, sat regally

on a Louis XVI throne, said, "You've made me look *so* fabulous; you *must* join me for a picture. Come on, hurry!"

I stood behind her.

Without turning her head to look at me, she said sharply, "*What* are you doing? *I* can't have you looking down on *me!* If you want your photograph taken with me, I suggest you *kneel!*"

I didn't even ask for a bloody photo, I thought, but you don't disobey the Iron Lady...

I'd got a print of it, had it framed and hung it in my living-room. Last week, some shag I brought home lectured me for having her on my wall.

"Did you come here for sex an' drugs or for a political debate? I'm not taking it down, so if you don't like it, fuck off!" I said, chopping lines of coke, and – to rephrase one of Maggie's speeches – as I wasn't in the mood to be fucked, added, "By the way, *this* puff's not for turning; *you* turn if you want to."

So he did, and I fisted him under Maggie's nose...

★★★★

My colour-code stickers – blue for cocaine, green for ketamine – were muddily identical in *Fist*'s crimson light. Nor could I differentiate lemon tranquilisers from off-white ecstasies with any certainty. I was playing Russian roulette, and I only knew for sure that I'd picked K when...

"YOU THINK YOU'RE SO DAMNED CLEVER, DON'T YOU?" said Mom as clearly as if I was fifteen.

157

…my muscles went leaden marshmallow, powerless to extricate a pumping dick and jaws on mine and fingers yanking my nipples…

"AIDAN, STOP HIM!" There it was again…

…the abdominal flutter of an unintentional Love Dove…

"Something I should've had twelve years ago," I heard Mom like I was back in 1980.

…the impotency which would irregularly accompany ecstasy and may in a little while rear its flaccid head alleviated with an unmistakable diamond-shaped Viagra…

"Scrub that muck off, you look like a bloomin' clown!" ordered Mom.

…the dirtiest acts to purge the past, cruising from man to man on E's loveable wings…

"Wanna bump of MDMA?" a charitable hunk asked.

I keenly accepted four untried letters to add to the alphabet of Class A's anaesthetising my system.

"You're a Brummie! I'm from Birmingham too," he said. We played list-the-clubs we used to go to and bartered a who's who of personages from our misspent youths – triggering in me remembrances of nigh on half a lifetime ago…that first line of cocaine I'd had…cat-fights under disco lights should any pretender purloin elements of my look…sleeping with Arthur just to see if he really did only have one testicle like my best friend The Very Miss Dusty O had said, then falling in love with Arthur when I'd discovered he had two and the despair I'd felt when it didn't develop into anything more… that first trip at The Kipper Club, and the chill-out afterwards at Gay John's bijou flat chock-a-block with more garish tat than Graceland, and the quickie we'd had which left me smiling like the cat who'd got the cream for a whole month after…

We established I didn't remember Chris. By his own admission he'd been but a peripheral player in those halcyon nights; he'd also lavished tens of thousands of pounds on a Ryan O'Neal face transplant. I'd less drastically but no less dramatically remodelled my shell by – after I'd upped sticks to London in '89 to follow my dream to be a make-up artist – chiselling off 5 kilos of *Chanel* cosmetics when I realised make-up made me look *more* like Mom, shearing off my Shakespear's Sister bob and ditching the hair dye too, and joining a gym and obsessively pumping iron until I'd expanded from a puny eight stone to a solid 176 lbs. My hard-earned pecs hung with nipple rings, and lats and biceps emphasised with Celtic tattoos, were a new form of drag as *de rigeur* to cut it in the '90s as being a New Romantic had been in the '80s. These days, I was 'Carl'.

"Did you know Stan?" asked Chris.

I played dumb – titillated to learn how I'd gone down in posterity.

"Strawberry Switchblade Stan," he said to jog my memory…

★★★★

Back in '85, fast-tracked through to meet the *'Since Yesterday'* songstresses, done up in their Siouxsie-meets-Liz-Taylor-meets-psychedelia look, the paparazzi had gone bananas…

'To Stan, Strawberry Switchblade's biggest fan,
Lots of Love Rose XXX'
'To Stan, Strawberry Switchblade's 3rd member,
you look great,
All My Love Jill XXXXX'

they'd written, vandalising my record sleeves with smilies and doodles of hearts and stars and their trademark hair bows…in next day's Birmingham Post above the caption **'Schoolboy meets sexy Switch singers at HMV signing'** a photo of me sandwiched between the real stars looking starrier than them…that crinkly page – along with all photographic proof of a history every bit as embarrassing as admitting to ever having been a Toyah fan – long ago consigned to the bin…

****

"You know, *Stan* – Stan who Titchy Pete gave a pearl necklace to."

Droll as it was to hear a Chinese whisper which had recast Wolverhampton Mark and distorted facts, I definitely had no awareness of *that* Stan.

"Stan with the flowers and the bird in his hair, wore a pink ball-gown, the best make-up in Birmingham, Stan who used to fall in love with someone different every week and bombard 'em with roses an' his last Rolo."

I'd done something similar at Infants, shaving Mom's dining-table centrepiece of crepe-paper blooms and bestowing them to girls on an unremitting quest for affection in the aftermath of Mom's…

"AIDAN, STOP HIM!" God, not again…

"Stan was the one who was obsessed with Linus."

I still was. Forty-eight seasons of heartache interspersed with two magical shags, glimmers of what *still* might be if only he'd commit himself, Linus was the one bygone I couldn't purge. That L-word was a preventative to lasting love elsewhere. *"There's this guy who's the love of my life and if he asks me out I'll say yes"* weren't exactly words to reassure those who were ready to affirm that theirs was unconditional...

"AIDAN, STOP HIM!"

I walked away on Chris mid-sentence...casting my net farther afield to climes where foreigners wouldn't exhume unwelcome ghosts – to Barcelona, to Miami, to Paris, to Cape Town, to Rome, to Amsterdam, to Ibiza – partying and whoring around the world in eighty gays through the mid-nineties, then diving back into the London club circuit with a vengeance in August, '97...

"DODI'S DEAD AND DIANA'S IN A COMA," squawked the Jamaican loon in luminous lime hot pants and co-ordinating bra and wig and lashes and Baby Spice-style platform trainers, running in figure-of-eights around Brixton Road's 24-hour Tesco forecourt. She was the pinnacle of an uproarious night spent snorting sufficient K to kill twenty horses and triple-dropping enough E to orbit the globe.

Laughing at her till we were hoarse and ennui set in, dazedly spent, the four of us staggered back to mine. To restart the party I put on Tatjana's Eurodisco floor-filler, *'Santa Maria'*, which had creamed us to extra-sensory overload on the dancefloor of *Love Muscle*, with its accompanying blizzard of silver ticker tape and pink balloons and pyrotechnics. Bank Richard organized drinks; Melinda, a part-time Bette Midler tribute act, racked up our pooled remnants of coke and ketamine, a confection she chicly labelled CK One after the *Calvin Klein* perfume; Drew, an ebony Schwarzenegger I'd nicknamed Diana Ross and The Supremes owing to his Miss Ross facial mannerisms and pneumatic pectorals which he could jiggle at will, had temporarily gone grey as he did when twatted, was horizontal on one sofa watching an empty screen. I turned the telly on so his dilated pupils would have something to watch…

"THAT MAD BITCH WASN'T MAD!" I said, thinking *Mom always said Princess Di was a car crash waiting to happen.*

Call the dealer, it's what Diana would've wanted was the group consensus. Once reinforcements arrived, we paid our respects until we were so high that sleep wouldn't be an option till Tuesday at the soonest…

"Let's go to *Trade*" – an after-hours dance asylum for insomniacs – "Diana would want us to. She loved the gays. The time she spent in an' out of The Lighthouse" – a hospice for AIDS patients – "anyone'd think *she* had it," said Drew.

In the taxi, as we pulled up alongside a refuse truck at an intersection, I jested, "I wonder which vehicle's got more trash in it, this one or that one?" Our driver, po-faced, retorting, "This one."

…*Trade*'s oxygen a smog of pheromones and sherbet-scented dry ice and amyl nitrate…the drug dealer's identity masked in a latex cartoon pig's head…the beats harder…the flicker-flash of high-tech lasers dehumanising faceless physiques all pulsating sexily to Hard House to freeze-frame robotics…leant against a wall coming up on E, next to me was a travesty, a hybrid of Linford Christie and Lolo Ferrari, her hairpiece secured with a headscarf knotted under her chin, lolloping forehead-to-the-wall to take the weight off her melon boobs...

"What's your name?" I asked.

"Elle," she drawled, American.

"Like the letter?"

"No, honey: the magazine."

"Are they real?"

"Sure are honey, they're a gift from God."

...my jeans getting soaked when a breast – Elle had over-estimated the resilience of an overtaxed condom – exploded...

"JUMP IN, STAN!"

...Did someone just shout 'Jump in, Stan'?

"ST-A-A-AN, HELLO-OH, EARTH CALLIN'! JUMP IN!" hollered Julie Bedwell, tugging me back to reality. It was 1984. She was floating on her back, her braless tits bobbing like buoys, in an Edwardian public baths which, today, wasn't public. There was neither *hoi polloi* nor personnel to dampen the spirits of Nick, Nicole, Jennifer, Gay John and Whiskers and his boyfriend, sprawled on slatted loungers smoking and drinking, bantering raucously...

"NO, I CAN'T SWIM!" I shouted.

Jah Wobble torpedoed by, alerting me to the potential peril of wearing non-waterproof make-up poolside, and I shielded my soluble face with my skirt as he dive-bombed Julie, sheltering myself 'til every last splish-splash had subsided, peeping over my skirt and... *Whoosh!*

"You what?" said Bank Richard.

We were slumped against the DJ booth.

"I said *I can't swim.*"

"Oh, that's what I thought you said."
"Where are we? What year is it?"
"Dunno."

A dancer beside us solved the conundrum:
"You're at *DTPM*, it's 1997."
"How did we get here?" I asked the dancer.
"I don't know, I've never met you before," he said, and danced away.
Richard shoved his K-bullet up my nostril.

> *'Oh, runaway, you better not hesitate,*
> *better hurry don't wait now, runaway'*

belted the diva, surfing on a crest of shimmery strings.

I sniffed hard…time evaporated…suddenly aware that…

"AIDAN, STOP HIM!"

…the Filter Disco hustle had sped up to 140bpm so I wasn't at *DTPM* anymore…

> *'He never lost his hardcore'*

intoned a voice deep in the mix…

How did I get here?

I was at after-after-aferhours club *FF.* No Richard, no Melinda, no Drew…

Turfed out of *FF* at 8 a.m. on a Monday, my t-shirt lost and almost my mind, the street meat-market was my last chance to cop off. I fell into the mouth of a wickedly charming Spanish acquaintance. Juan Carlos was the father of last Saturday's juvenile sexploit. He'd moved back to Spain, and was here on holiday. After a year-long long-distance love affair, I relinquished my glittering make-up career and emigrated to a torpid life in Sevilla paid for by the rent from my Stockwell flat, a flat paid off by a premature inheritance from Dad. Baring my soul to Juan Carlos, he counseled, "She's no mother. You should sever all ties with her," so I rang her to tell her.....

"Why?" she cried.

Even though I hadn't quite pieced the fragments together myself, I replied, "You know why," and hung up…his domination and my narcotic paranoia soon curdling our *Te quiero* to thirteen months of *TE ODIO* 'til all there was left to express was whiskey violence.... returning to Blighty at the close of the millennium…

After I'd vomited up a bad E – over a stranger's shoulder whilst watching the NYE fireworks on Victoria Embankment – once I was re-toxed I had an explosive start to Y2K, drug-fucked and fucking through the Kama Sutra with a between-letdown-boyfriends fuck-buddy with caramel skin, curly black hair, and a bubble-butt and Duracell dick to die for – the happily-ever-after that might've been had I not liked him too much to hang my hang-ups on him, or had faith he wouldn't hang *his* on me…resurrecting my career then hopping back on the drugs`n`clubs merry-go-round, on a hunt for the Holy Grail…bedding roses but waking up with weeds, if I was incapable of rescuing me then I'd rescue them…

"AIDAN, STOP HIM!"

165

…only their fragility would foster mine. An Italian lapdog; a K-dealing drain; a steroid hothead; and a Kiwi clam who in eighteen months never once took his Stussy cap off even to perform fellatio, its peak still indented in my abdomen eighteen months after we'd unshackled ourselves. When those relationships failed to be *yang* to my *yin* there'd be irrational showdowns and ferocious recriminations – replays of Simon, visions of Mom's mascara cesspools…

"AIDAN, STOP HIM!"

Tired of princes who'd turn into frogs – me *and* them – fuck *Mills & Boon*…muddling from druggy one-night-stand to druggy one-night-stand, my sexual partners into quadruple figures…drug consumption spiralling. The tawdry glamour of sharing yesterday's hero Steve Strange's makeshift crack-pipe – a brown-stained Evian bottle with a biro tube lanced through one side – in a shitty cubicle in *Crash* nightclub. How far he'd fallen but how far I'd risen!

"Hey, I'm gonna be doing the *Here and Now Tour*. I'm gonna be playing Newcastle, Sheffield, Bournemouth, Cardiff, Brighton, Birmingham and Manchester," croaked Steve between puffs, in a slo-mo voice like he'd been gargling gravel all his life. "I can't pay you much but I'd love you to be my make-up artist."

"Well, cuz it's you I'll do it for fifty quid a show plus expenses," I said.

"Expenses?" he asked.

"Yeah, there'll be hotel and travel costs."

"*Nooooo*, I've already arranged to cadge a lift in The Belle Stars' mini-bus, they're lovely girls, they won't mind if I bring you too."

Chugging the length and breadth of the UK cramped in

a ten-seater with Steve, his crack-pipe, and seven butch girls plus instruments rehearsing 'Iko Iko' could only be a magical *misery* tour which, by tour's end, with my addictive personality I could see I'd be a crack addict too. 'Fade To Grey'.

Thanks, but no thanks, I'll stick to coke, E, K, LSD and MDMA, I thought.

Cavernous comedowns made bleaker by *'Torment & Toreros'* which was crueller in its remastered CD clarity, a thumb-sucking forever fourteen...

"AIDAN, STOP HIM!"

A knackered, come-drenched, coke-addled cadaver, albeit one whose shell – thanks to Peter Pan genes and *Clinique Turn-around Cream* – gave the lie of health...whose hereditary work ethic had for two decades obligated him to never miss a day's work...although, nudging forty, it was increasingly draining to burn the candle at both ends...quarter-hourly amphetamine dabs on the job just to stay afloat, nostrils permanently powder-crusted, stone-cold sweats in midsummer, tropical perspiration in midwinter...

"AIDAN, STOP HIM!"

All the coke and all the cocks didn't hold the key...
"Enough's enough...unless you want what for"...enough depravity for infinite reincarnations...eschewing dissipation for celibate introspection through the looking glass of Narcotics Anonymous and hypnotherapy...

"When I was a teenager..." I blamed her...
"When you were a teenager..." she blamed me...

167

Our shouty slam-the-receiver-downs an impasse to reparation, our uncommunicative intervals ever-lengthened... I was regressing back-back-back, to a pitiful six-year-old, bereft and guilty. *"Embrace that inner child, love him,"* advised my hypnotherapist, Sean.

Putting pen to paper, mapping out my life in a little book of sorrows and, in my lucid solitude, jigsawing together the shards of that nightmarish childhood episode, why I had throughout these drug-diet years been hearing myself beg "AIDAN, STOP HIM!" shone phosphorescent...

12

'So goodbye, yellow brick road...'

Elton John

1976.

"Hi love! Sorry I'm late!"

"Don't 'love' me. Isn't the factory 'phone working? You think I've got nothing better to do than wait around for you? Especially with *them* whining they're hungry every two seconds like they're bloody Cambodians! And *this*'ll be inedible," harrumphed Mom, reaching into the oven.

"That's alright, love, I'm not fussy," answered Dad blithely, as if Mom was apologising for overcooked faggots, chips and peas, and dodging the flying plate just in time…

"What was *that* for?"

That was the second wrong thing Dad could've said. A cue for Aidan and me to make a sharp exit, and Mom's cue to throw a loud lengthy catalogue of grievances in his face…

"I ONLY MARRIED YOU TO ESCAPE MY FAMILY AN' I'VE BEEN SACRIFICING MYSELF SINCE! AND I'LL *NEVER* FORGIVE YOU FOR CONSENTING TO ELECTRIC SHOCK THERAPY!"

"What's electric shock therapy?" I asked. Aidan shrugged.

"You can't blame me, love! That was the doctor's – "

"QUIET! I'M TALKING! I MEAN, *WHAT* LOVING HUSBAND IN HIS RIGHT MIND WOULD AGREE TO *THAT*?"

A second plate smashed against the tiles…

"JAN, STOP!"

"STOP?! I HAVEN'T BLOODY STARTED! I CAN'T TAKE ANY MORE OF THIS! YOU *NEVER* DO YOUR SHARE WITH THE BLOODY KIDS, KIDS *I* NEVER WANTED IN THE FIRST PLACE! GOD, EVERYTHING THAT'S WRONG IN MY LIFE IS *YOUR* FAULT! DON'T JUST STAND THERE, YOU PILLOCK. SAY SOMETHING!"

"I've been trying, but – "

A third plate…

"SHUT UP! AND I CAN'T BELIEVE THAT WHEN DAD DIED" – Billy had had a fatal heart attack at work – "*YOU* THOUGHT THAT GOING BACK TO THE BLOODY FACTORY WAS MORE IMPORTANT THAN WAITING HERE TO TELL ME YOURSELF! I HAD TO HEAR IT FIFTH-HAND FROM A COLLEAGUE! WHAT HAVE YOU GOT TO SAY ABOUT *THAT*?"

"I didn't know where you were or what time you'd be home…I said I was sorry…you know I love you, Jan – "

"LOVE, THAT'S A BLOODY JOKE! YOU DON'T KNOW THE MEANING OF THE WORD! I SHOULD'VE LISTENED TO DAD!"

170

"Mom's coming," Aidan and I said in unison, and split to our rooms.

Hearing a crashing thud and a fraught clitter-clatter, I tiptoed in to observe Mom strong-arming the contents of her extensive wardrobe – all still on its hangers – into the suitcase she'd heaved from its top.

"What're you doing, Mom?"

She didn't answer. Sitting on the case and snapping it shut, she pushed through me as though I were invisible, and struggled downstairs with me in pursuit hectoring, "Where're we going? Can I get my dolls?" She strained to cram it into the boot of her Triumph Spitfire, barked, "GET OUT OF MY WAY!" and backed down the driveway at speed.

"MOM, DON'T GO!"

Dad, waking up to the fact that she'd gone, sprinted to his Citroën GS, and with neither a bye nor leave, disappeared into the yonder. Parentless, we huddled together on the porch step, stoical Aidan doing his utmost to console me, disconsolate as I was. His assurances that Dad would bring her home were dashed when only one car returned. Dad – not showing the slightest disturbance at our anguish, chirpily saluting Gail and Pete from next-door who were on their way out – shepherded us indoors…

Janet was too angry for tears – driving aimlessly, blaspheming at drivers beeping at her, swerving from lane to lane – heedless of give way signs or red lights. One hour later, she pulled over to gather her thoughts. *I wish Dad was alive, he'd understand why I left. Why didn't I listen to you, Dad? Marrying John when you could see I shouldn't have… Why did you have to die when we were just beginning to get to know each other?*

★★★★

"Where's Mom?" Janet had asked that day last summer, knowing full well Winnie wouldn't do two buses, and wouldn't come if Janet didn't drive the twenty mile round trip to pick her up.

"Oh, you know..." Billy sighed without elaborating – father and daughter mindful not to badmouth Winnie in front of Aidan and Carl who were affectionately annihilating their granddad like untrained Great Danes.

"Well it's her loss," said Janet. "Let's make the most of it. C'mon Dad, I'll show you 'round."

Billy Fletcher, an uneducated man who still slogged fifty hour weeks for minimum salary, could never have dreamt of this – a detached house with two lounges and a laundry room and three garages – for himself *or* his progeny.

"I'm so proud of you and what all your hard work's achieved," he beamed. Though Janet had long yearned for her dad's praise, her mind was elsewhere... How much slighter he seemed in these spacious rooms than in his matchbox maisonette; how much older than sixty he looked against the up-to-date décor of brash primary patterns pared-down by neutral browns – Janet's interpretation of the glossy aspirations in *Ideal Homes* magazine.

"You used to love your allotment, didn't you? You're going to love the garden," she said, theatrically pulling up the vertical blind on the sliding patio doors to unveil thirty feet of flora and fauna. She helped him navigate the step down. As Billy paused to admire the dozen varieties of rose, the rhododendron bush, peonies, fuchsias and purple clematis which were all blooming marvellous in early summer; the

172

vegetable patch that was a luscious medley; and the chicken coop – his craggy face lit up, and a wave of delight overcame her.

Janet went to make a pot of tea. Sat on the bench below the weeping willow, Billy reviewed the idyllic vista – a Shangri-La he couldn't allow himself to relish fully. He had an inkling things weren't quite as rosy as they appeared. Which had nothing to do with Carl, six, gambolling on the lawn in a hydrangea chiffon gown; or Aidan, nine, vivisecting a toad by the pond; or the fact that the coop was a scene of feathery carnage after foxes – sensing a succulent feast – massacred the chickens the previous night.

"Are you happy, Jan?"

"AIDAN, DON'T HIT CARL! WHAT? CAROLINE, STOP PROVOKING HIM! AND AIDAN, STOP RISING TO THE BAIT! God, I wish I never had them sometimes! Of course I'm happy, why wouldn't I be?"

Her curt denial was as much to satisfy herself as him...

"Remember what I said to you on your wedding day?"

Those fleeting moments in the limousine back in 1961 were the only time they'd been alone 'til now.

"Well, it's still not too late."

"Whaddya mean *it's not too late*?"

She knew exactly what he was inferring though...

Billy rested his hand on Janet's – an insignificant gesture to most but a momentous one coming from this man whose mother had died when he was four; coming from a father she couldn't recall ever being tactile. She desperately wanted to say *'I love you'*, but as she'd never told him and couldn't

173

imagine it not sticking in her gullet she settled on momentarily resting her other hand on his. Then the awkwardness of intimacy made her release her hands, pour more tea, and pilot the conversation back to the safer ground of superficialities…

When she volunteered to chauffeur him home, Billy declined. "You've got enough on your plate here, Jan. And John'll be back soon, you'll have to start getting dinner on the go. No, I'll be fine. I've had a wonderful afternoon; I'll remember it as long as I live. And remember what I said Johnuck."

That had been his pet name for her way back when. Hearing it, she smiled so her cheeks ached; she'd cry if antidepressants would allow it. She watched him shuffle to the end of the path, Carl flanking him, begging, "Don't go, Granddad", and she knew that no matter what had gone unsaid, today was a cornerstone on which they'd build something more profound.

★★★★

"Fifty years stuck in a crappy sweatshop when you loved the countryside, thirty-five years stuck in an even crappier marriage…why didn't I tell you I love you? I'm sorry, I'm sorry," she sobbed, hammering her forehead on the steering-wheel, mourning his wasted life, leaching savage tears which no tablets could defeat…

She hadn't cried 'til now, hadn't had time to.

Winnie had nominated Janet to arrange the funeral. *You're brainier than our Linda, and your brothers couldn't organize a piss-up in a brewery*, she'd said, a sly dig to berate Billy's boozing. And Janet hadn't cried graveside, or at the wake when if nobody actually spoke ill of the deceased they didn't speak well of him either – nobody bounding to Billy's defence when his boss told Janet, "I didn't believe your dad when he boasted his eldest daughter was a teacher living in a big house in a posh area."

"I *hope* you're not insinuating my father was a liar – he was worth a million of you," she'd snapped, to the consternation of the Fletcher clan whose unquestionable attitude to holders of authority was cap-doffing. But she wasn't cut from the same sackcloth as them, and had indignantly shown him the door. She'd have to deal with her grief another day, another week, another month…

Bringing her face up to the rear-view mirror, pain colouring her features more effectively than *Estée Lauder* ever could, Janet stared longer than she should. She was scared; scared because she hadn't seen this reflection – the hollow manifestation of depression – since Carl was a baby. *I don't want this fucking life, kids and a useless fucking husband and a fulltime job I don't get a thank-you for… Expensive clothes and handbags, cars and holidays abroad, what's it all for? I'm no better off than Dad… I can't go on like this, the same old crap year-in year-out 'til I die… What's the bloody point in living?*

In that instant, she made her decision, and – calm and serene, and complying with the Highway Code – she made her way home.

"Stop crying Carl, she'll have to come back sooner or later. And when she does, don't you two go upsetting her," said Dad as if it'd been *us* who'd been late for dinner, *us* who'd inflamed her. We nodded, gawping at a TV that didn't amuse but whose fluttering pixels and droning tone provided distraction.

The eventual vibration of Mom's engine stirred us from our stupor and we rushed to welcome her. Looking less than her ordinarily impeccable self, like an uncoloured-in line drawing with her make-up all cried off, she dumped her suitcase, pushed us away, and said, "I'm going to bed, I don't wanna be disturbed." As impenetrable as she was, at least now she was home, there were no screeching arguments or thrown crockery, and we could enjoy what was left of *Fawlty Towers*…

She counted to sixty. Any doubts she had about what she had in mind were tempered when John didn't come after her. Okay, she'd said not to but she still expected him to, even at the risk of having his fucking head bitten off. She counted to sixty again, John's foghorn laughter filtering through the floorboards.

I'll have the last laugh, you won't be laughing when you have to work fulltime and raise them yourself…

She lay down to be reunited with Billy, departing this mortal coil so effortlessly…

"Bedtime, Carl. Check on your mom, will you? If she's sleeping don't wake her up though, you don't wanna make her angry."

I entered the room as cautiously as possible. She was dead to the world, a streak of streetlight highlighting the contours of her fully-clothed body. I crept out, hung over the banister, and yelled "SHE'S FAST ASLEEP!" so loud the whole neighbourhood knew. Cuddling my *Holly Hobbie* rag doll, I floated off to sleep dreaming of cloudless tomorrows full of cuddles and hundreds-and-thousands-sprinkled *Angel Delight* and puppies…shaken awake by Dad shouting, "WHY DIDN'T YOU SAY SHE'S TAKEN AN OVERDOSE?"

"A *what?* Stop it, Dad, you're hurting me!"

But he wouldn't let up, shaking me harder and harder 'til my cries woke Aidan.

"Dad, what's happening?" he asked.

"SHUT UP AIDAN! CALL 999, ASK FOR AN AMBULANCE...*NOW!*"

Still Dad didn't stop shaking me, warning, "PRAY YOUR MOM SURVIVES – 'CAUSE IF SHE DOESN'T..."

"WHAT DID I DO? STOP! AIDAN, STOP HIM! AIDAN, PLEASE!"

Suddenly our house was abuzz with uniformed strangers whose abrupt intrusion – scary though it initially was – was a blessed relief when Dad let go of me.

"Go to your rooms boys, this isn't for children's eyes," said one kindly man, as another fed tubing down Mom's throat, and two others busied themselves with monitoring apparatus, the parental bedroom resembling the set of *Angels*...

Next I knew it was the morning after the nightmare before. Things were almost as if nothing had happened, except Dad chivvied us to get ready for school; Mom had no make-up on and her hair wasn't coiffed; Dad drove me to school and picked me up; and that evening Mom was still a pallid scarecrow and Dad cooked tea.

For a short while John pulled his weight but it didn't last...

How the hell will I handle depression now? 'Cause Dr McEvoy won't prescribe tablets again, fretted Janet.

She didn't mean to be violent but sometimes she just couldn't help herself, and venting her fury – giving the kids 'what for' – did always seem to help...

Mom's unpredictable 'what fors' were way scarier than the nightmares that plagued me for a long, long time after. Her leaving home in a huff lugging her suitcase didn't distress me anymore. It was her homecomings which distressed me, having to walk on eggshells, loins girded for her next 'what for'....

13

'Freedom comes when you learn to let go...'

'The Power of Goodbye' Madonna

Aidan never fulfilled Janet's Uni dream. He'd dropped out after half a term, dossed around for a bit and then found work as a road-labourer. So much for investing a fortune on his education... Like everything else in her life, it seemed if she wanted it she'd have to do it herself, so in 1987 she gave up work to do a degree in Psychology.

It was ironic that her scholarly clique – with all their psychoanalytic nous and certificates coming out their ears – looked at her fairy-tale mansion, her *à la mode* finery, and her Prince Charming husband and thought she had it all. It was ironic because the only soul to ever see through her subterfuge was Billy who hadn't a qualification to his name. Ironic, because even as she'd been digesting her lecture notes on *'The Lying Brain: An Examination Of Hallucinations And Delusions In The Normal, Clinical and Pathological Population'* and Billy had come to her prodding *It's still not too late* she still kidded herself... Ironic, because even as she'd bawled at Carl, "WE WON'T BE HAPPY 'TIL YOU GO!" – something she'd done daily in the three years before he'd left home – in her heart-of-hearts she'd known it wasn't so. Carl's transgressions – another two shoplifting convictions; nabbing him nicking money from them God knows how many more times; astronomical 'phone bills; vermillion hair dye in the grouting and peroxide spillages on the landing carpet; incessant disruptive music; crashing her car; bringing men back – were all she and John had really talked about.

She'd long ago grown accustomed to John's thousand-yard stare in response to her scintillating monologues, yet she'd always been all-ears-responsive to his repetitive golf-tennis-factory-golf drivel; but as she got more intellectual stimulation the more she glazed over too when he prattled on. *He's not gonna change* she'd think, too dispirited for conflict or plate-hurling, and she'd traipse to the dining-room and dig around in the sideboard drawer that was the family archive. She dug out her press-cuttings:

'Embroidery? Janet prefers engineering'

read one, reporting on *'pert, pretty and as smart as they come'* Janet Fletcher, the teenage aspiring mechanic with *'a smudge of grease on her nose'* who'd been awarded a ten-guinea cheque for her distinction in mathematics.

'Young wife wins trip abroad'

read another, apprising readers that Mrs Janet Stanley, 21, had won ten days at an international youth conference in Germany for being GKN's star apprentice and best all-round young employee. She studied old photos: a heavily pregnant bouffant-ed blimp in a bar in Tenerife pouring vino blanco down her neck from one of those point-spouted jugs; another rocking week-old Carl in her arms, simulating joyfulness for the camera but her concave face zombie-eyed; one of an ingénue, just seventeen, just engaged, looking more like a widow than a fiancée; a timid bride, gripping on to the ribbon-reins of four horseshoes, talismans to assuage her she hadn't signed away more than her maiden name. She'd spend many a lunchtime in the University's Barber Institute of Fine Art admiring the Pre-Raphaelites' beatific impressions of milestones in women's lives, but writ large in the pictures of her life she saw the emotions those artists had chosen not to paint...

Seminars on the function of neurons; on variations in human and animal psychology; on statistical analysis, and the processes of associative learning – and even those on consumer behaviour and child behaviour and the assessment and treatment of mental illness, three modules which shouldn't have been quite so knotty for a shopaholic diagnosed-depressive one-time-lithium-taker electroshocked mother of miscreants – may have taxed her to her limits by day, but far more troubling was the recurring horror infiltrating her nights. Bugs crawled all over her, under her eyelids and inside her mouth, gorging on her like she was buried alive. She'd swat, scratch and spit all night, and awake exhausted, with self-inflicted lacerations and an ulcerated tongue. Janet didn't need Jung to unravel what this meant; she just needed to heed Billy's words. Otherwise, overdosing on tedium would be an excruciatingly slow suicide…

When she told John, in a histrionic outburst one Saturday afternoon in a rammed pub in Covent Garden, she'd cried wolf so many times he thought she was joking.

Even when the removal van came, he didn't believe it.

Two sofas, her *Lladro*, a jardinière, her clothes, her make-up and her *Braun Independent Cordless Style'n' Go* were all she took to her modest new semi. But she wasn't any happier, and the compulsory therapy she had to submit to as part of her post-grad counsellor training only extracted more anger that she'd squandered three decades on John, more sadness about her upbringing...

★★★★

In the middle of World War II, having stomped out on her husband-of-one-year well into her third trimester, Winnie had gone into labour at her mom and dad's. Some who knew her might claim that the real reason Winnie had had difficulty forcing the baby out herself was that she was bone idle, but those who *had* been present could attest that forceps weren't an easy ride. As the midwife stretched her with the torturous steel contraption and clamped the crown stuck in her cervix, passers-by who'd heard the howls emanating from an upper-storey window and paused outside the poor-but-proud terrace wondered if they were eavesdropping on manslaughter. Only when those screams were overwhelmed by a babe's could they go about their business safe in the knowledge they'd heard a painful delivery, nothing more.

Once weary Winnie had got her breath back and been stitched up, the midwife told her the left side of her 10lbs whopper of a daughter's face was paralysed, warning Winnie that if it wasn't massaged every hour on the hour the paralysis would be permanent. There was absolutely no way Winnie had the patience to nurse Janet, so her snap-decision, to leave Granny holding the baby and go about *her* business – back to Billy to give it another go – was a blessing in disguise. Well, almost.

Winnie's absence meant mother and daughter didn't bond, and even after Janet was fully recovered and Winnie reclaimed her, they never did – any affection Winnie might have had for the child who'd caused her such pain, or a husband to whom she was so woefully mismatched, transferred instead to her second daughter who slipped painlessly into being.

It had always rankled with Janet that Linda was Winnie's golden girl…

★★★★

All those times Winnie had grumbled *'Stop wasting your bloody time reading, there's housework that needs doing'*, and yet when Janet had got into grammar school Winnie would brag about it like it'd been down to her! And Billy choosing ale over her throughout her childhood still aggrieved her even now, although it was a dead cert it had been Winnie – who'd always use his absences to intoxicate the kids with poisonous comments about what a pathetic specimen he was – who he'd been escaping. They were undemonstrative parents, undemonstrative spouses too. Janet hadn't ever seen them touch, let alone kiss. That they'd procreated three times was miraculous, and by the time Winnie fell pregnant for the fourth time, at forty-three, it must've been an immaculate conception as she and Billy didn't even *talk*. Mortified though Winnie was when the pregnancy was confirmed, it did have its perks: it was an excuse to sit down, gripe *'I can't cope'* over and over, and be mollycoddled for eight months.

Now, Janet had the tools to understand that Winnie had always done that with death too…

"I can't cope," Winnie said when Grandpa Jones died.

"Your poor mother, she couldn't cope when our Nelly died of chickenpox either," newly-widowed Granny Jones had said, cosseting her thirty-six-year-old daughter as if she was four again – while Winnie's brothers and sisters fussed over her too.

"I can't cope," Winnie said when Granny Jones died.

Forget that they were anybody else's losses, because nobody suffered bereavement like poor, poor Winnie!

It had narked Janet to watch her mother playact the distraught widow – a part she'd shammed to perfection, wailing *I can't cope* through barren tears while hosting callers who'd marvel *You're coping so well, Winnie.*

Janet wasn't so pitiless as to deny Winnie her right to be grief-stricken by Kev's death, but Winnie's was a tearless grief, guilt-ridden in the belief that his death was divine retribution for her not wanting him, and she sat down for a quarter of a century after that. Yes, she'd still worked at the *Speed Queen Laund-o-rama*, where she'd become manageress after Kev had begun Infants', but she'd sat down there too while Big Gladys and Winkie Gladys did all the work – the launderette a podium where the community came in day-in day-out to venerate her bravery, everybody choosing to forget that Kev had been the one with cancer, not speaking his name in case it demolished Winnie.

Nobody was any the wiser that Winnie's sphinx-like fortitude was the consequence of an addiction to prescription pills and that – like a sphinx – she couldn't emote beyond a passive smile.

"You'll regret leaving John, you won't find another good'un like him at your age," Winnie had censured. Grateful though Janet was that her mom had chipped in in her murkiest post-natal days, though it still needled her that Winnie had managed to juggle work with being a mother-of-sorts to Paul and Kev *and* child-mind newborn Carl, it needled her *more* that Winnie still thought the sun shone out of John's arse…

★★★★

1992, the Queen's *annus horribilis*, was Janet's *annus horribilis* too…turning fifty…stagnating in unhappy, loveless limbo… doubtful lately if John had really loved her given how briskly he'd embarked on a new liaison…doubtful if love would ever be hers. Those volumes of self-help tomes advocating *self-love through self-acceptance* which she'd insatiably gobble through her sleepless nights all pressed readers to delve deeper into their minds' for resolution, to seek professional guidance if necessary.

Janet knew that – whatever pain it might unleash – she *had* to do it if she was going to move on. She chose Rebirthing therapy, a branch of psychotherapy purporting to guide patients to the moment of delivery and professing *that* to be our blueprint for our life. Armed with facts galore about her birth, the ones Winnie had recited so often through the years, she set out to heal her life under the fatherly tutelage of her therapist, David.

Rebirthing allowed her to *feel* herself strangulated, smothered, fighting for breath, those forceps clamping her temples, her face numbed, and – after all the sobbing and trauma those sessions aroused – David's final analysis wasn't so earth-shattering: Janet's life had been a scuffle right from the get-go…

David also strove to instill in her the knowledge that she wasn't accountable for Winnie's emotional incapacity, or for Billy's, or for John's; that she couldn't blame them, or any other soul living or dead for who, why, how or where she was; that she was a human *being* not a human *doing*; that only by absolving her mind of anxieties past and future would she have tranquillity to be in the present.

Zen ideology was fine in theory but it wasn't so easy to put into practise.

Not when John filed for divorce on the grounds of unreasonable behaviour so he could wriggle out of divvying their chattels 50-50. Not when her settlement ended up being half the worth of their house and half John's business, which – as he was about to retire anyway - he'd lost interest in.

Not when she'd have to toil tirelessly to rebuild it, to make it profitable so it would afford her the nest egg she needed now she knew she wasn't entitled to a penny of their pensions and her dotage wouldn't be as luxurious as she'd forecast.

Not when she'd invest her heart in men who weren't her equals emotionally or academically and stay in those affairs well past their sell by date – just like she had with John – wasting weeks each time they bit the dust repenting the repetition of her old familiar wrongs.

Not when Carl blamed her for Lord-only-knows-what as if she'd been the worst mother since Joan Crawford, and in 1998 had told her by 'phone from Seville that she was good as dead to him – a pronouncement which had pierced her like a rusty dagger…

But Janet had rebuilt the business, sold it and banked a tidy profit; she was getting quicker at divesting herself of ill-suited suitors; and blood had proved thicker than water because, once that dreadful Spanish shit-stirrer – possibly Spain's revenge on England over Gibraltar – was out of the frame, she and Carl had reconciled. Although their reconciliation hung by a thread when the disputes they had about politics or monarchy were prone to plummet into mutual condemnation:

Janet weepily bewailing, "You've no idea how hard my life's been!" and Carl irritably retaliating, "Course I fucking know! I'm sick of fucking hearing about it! If you were half as good a fucking listener as you are a talker, you'd know how hard *my* fucking life's been!"

Five years down the line, however, Carl was on his own voyage of self-healing. Sharing the philosophies they'd acquire from New Age handbooks, they became more empathic, mellower and more magnanimous. There was a genuine amity, something Janet regretted she hadn't had with her mom or dad, and could never forge with her mom now…

14

'All the hurt can be healed...'

'*Falling*' Kylie Minogue

Alzheimer's at last gave Nan the ultimate ruse to sit down. She'd make her body – as slim as it had been before gestation had ruined her waistline – such a deadweight that lifting her up out of her chair was a mammoth three-man task it was easier not to bother with. Her inert leg muscles had all but packed in, though her doctor said she had the constitution of an ox with the stamina to climb Mount Everest if she'd put her mind to it. She didn't have to do *anything* for herself now, and she was in her element.

She was clueless she'd had children. She'd ask hers

Who are you?

and titter at their replies, *I'm your son* or *I'm your daughter*, and if Aidan or I said, *I'm your grandson*, she'd belly laugh like she hadn't since before Kev died. One day, she was adamant I was Granddad; she irately knocked the spoon I was feeding her with from my hand, simmering "You're a vile man, Billy. Why did I marry you?"

It was fantastic to see a spark of her long-dormant pluck, for in her prime the Nan I preferred to recall – not this unkempt stranger, or insensate Nan, or Mom's bitter collage of her mother – had been a titanium-beehive broad who ruled the *Speed Queen* like she was Holloway Prison's top dog; the muggers and burglars who'd prowl Windmill Lane Precinct never violated her premises or person; charity service washes and teas and coffees were offered for those in dire financial straits; there was bawdy repartee with her male patrons.

That beehive which had been her greatest achievement had long since gone – not because her follicles had given up the ghost too, but because, even nearing ninety, Nan's hair was so profuse that the care home's mobile hairdresser had taken it upon herself to save herself undue aggro and give Nan an unglamorously manageable crop.

"Our Billy doesn't like darkies, do you? Look at that fat'un over there, I wouldn't do his job for all the tea in China," said Nan – alluding to the African momma across the dayroom sponging up a dandelion lake of urine. "Ooh, what am I going to do if they all want a cuppa tea? I don't have enough cups… d'you want pasteurized or sterilized milk in your tea?"

Mom and I shared a smile; humour was our mechanism for coping with Nan's condition. Each time we visited, I'd enter and re-enter the dayroom, and Nan would greet me on every occasion like I was a different visitor. Often there'd be a glint in her eyes as if she was in on the joke – the same girlish glint she'd have whenever she hid her false teeth and watched us search for them in every nook and cranny – shades of that princess who'd let everybody else run around after her.

"So, do you want me to type up this book you're writing?" asked Mom, feeding Nan with little more success now that Nan had receded to the faraway era between the wars where her Alzheimer's mostly left her, thinking Mom was her mother and playing silly buggers and refusing to eat. With her line-less face, it was easy to picture Nan as a little girl.

Mom had already offered her typing skills last year but I'd refused – more from discomfort at the thought of her reading about the extent of a drug intake which I hadn't quite admitted to myself yet than to protect her feelings. But this time, being a Luddite who'd never even *looked* at a computer, not only did I say yes, I asked her to contribute an afterword too. It would be the postscript to our bonding process, I thought.

It wasn't.

All I got was a series of vitriolic answerphone messages listing my 'lies' one-by-one, Mom's answerphone every time I'd ring her, and direct-to-voicemail if I called her mobile…

Through Aidan's intervention she *did* start picking up the 'phone again, but ours were cat-and-mouse exchanges at best, and frequently degenerated to virulent allegations of filial betrayal. Mom might have said that she understood my book was, at heart, a positive tale of two dented souls pining for love and understanding – characters who happened to be us – that she wanted to be part of, but as long as I suspected there was a shred of self-pitying defensiveness on her part, *I* didn't want her to be a part of it…

By then, she'd mailed me back the score of A4 jotters my pen-calloused knuckles had filled, and I'd bought a laptop and was blistering my fingertips addictively transcribing them day and night. But I wasn't tech-savvy, I didn't know about *'CTRL S'*, or *'File'*, or *'Save As'*, and inadvertently wiped my hard drive along the way.

Data recovery failed to recoup my unsaved document.

What? You're telling me you can catch Pete Townshend but you can't find 45,000 words?

Five hundred quid spunked down the drain and all my spontaneous prose lost in cyberspace. I persevered, compulsively hitting *'CTRL S', 'File'* and *'Save As'*, emailing it to myself, conscientiously storing it on two USB Keys.

I was typing when the caller ID flashed *'INTERNATIONAL'.*

Mom was holidaying in Almeria. At 6 a.m. I knew it was her, and why she was 'phoning. Sitting upright breathing had become too much effort for Nan.

In light of the on-going tension between me and Mom, I went to the funeral with Dad. I hadn't allowed her bias about his inadequacies to tarnish my relations with him in the way Nan had hers with Granddad. If I'd been in Dad's shoes *I'd* have sanctioned ECT too, *and* I'd have flung a few plates back at her, and – irrespective of his previous paternal short-comings – at least *he* could say "I love you, son" these days. Mom and Dad didn't talk now…

The launderette had been boarded up sometime during John Major's premiership, and the martyred matriarch hadn't been a visible presence in the neighbourhood since around 9/11, but her former customers and neighbours, and the descendants of those whom she had outlived, and even mates of Kev's, were all out in force nonetheless – unrelated mourn-ers braving blustery rain and outnumbering Winifred Fletcher's sprawling bloodline four to one. This impressive turnout made it all the harder for Janet, designated to perform the family eulogy by her siblings who – their mother's children through and through – were too grief-stricken to envisage doing it themselves.

Improvising from her list of bullet-points, incorporating into her oration *'doting grandmother'* and *'generous to a fault'* in accordance with the time-honoured convention of deifying the dearly departed; adding a yarn about the time a panicked Winnie sent the precinct on a wild-goose chase when she thought eight-year-old Kev had been kidnapped only to find the tearaway hidden in a washer, only ever in danger of being boil-washed by Winnie; Janet's apprehension intensified as the positive stories dwindled. She'd guessed *'unaffectionate mother'* and *'clashing personalities'* would stun the congregation, that there'd be order-of-services rustling and clearing of throats and downcast gazes, but when she uttered the word 'forgive', her walls crumbled. She'd always been adept at self-restraint in public; now her tears stunned even her. It could've been me speaking at her memorial…

My eyes met Mom's. I was in tears.

The motorcade passed Nan's old maisonette on its way to the cemetery. I wondered if Beanpole Ray still lived there; last I'd heard he'd a sex change. The procession trickled up Windmill Lane where, as a child, I'd rambled so many Saturdays with Nan, Mom and Aidan prior to Kev's death, past the indoor market where Nan would indulge us with toys and sweets. I chortled, remembering that time in the late '70s, when – with tabloids predicting that the arrival on British soil of America's number one drug pandemic *Angel Dust* (coincidentally the name of a crackle-on-the-tongue sherbet) would cause death and destruction and turn this green and satanic land's problematic adolescents into crazed assassins – Nan had said *I saw that Angel Dust stuff that's in the papers in our newsagents. I'll buy some for you to try.*

On the mausoleums of the cemetery's richest inhabitants,

those moss-mottled apostles and oxidised angels soaring through the rolling mists seemed to hover majestically. It hadn't got properly light today. I remembered going to Granddad Stan's funeral dressed in that same black net cocoon I'd worn to run away to Bloxwich – a black net veil draped over my black beehive, black lipstick and black nail varnish – and thought how much more suitable *that* outfit would have looked in this weather than the brilliant sunshine there'd been that day…

While Billy Fletcher enjoyed eternal peace a hundred strides away, Nan – as per her wishes pre-dementia – was lowered into the grave where Uncle Kevin had lain undisturbed for twenty-six years. I was thinking I should have brought a can of *Elnett* hairspray to be buried with Nan – like Pharaohs were buried with their prized possessions to take to the afterlife – when Mom, her *Lancôme Flash Bronzer* faintly marbled, edged forward and tossed an olive branch onto the coffin.

Her forgiving Nan *once* had been astonishing, but *twice*? This wasn't the woe-is-me Mom I'd spent my entire life disliking even if, in adulthood, I esteemed her as a remarkable woman who'd clawed her way from relative poverty to be an engineer, a teacher, a shrewd businesswoman, and – latterly – a Labour councillor. Now that I'd learned to like myself flaws and all, now that I could appreciate those traits of hers I had inherited that I *liked* – her tenacity, her humour, her heart – if only she'd hold her hands up, admit that *my* perspective of the past wasn't the figment of a woe-is-me son's imagination then I'd give her a bloody olive grove and *like* her.

As I left the wake, she pressed an envelope into my hands, hugged me tight and said, "I love you."

I began to cry and fled…

Once I was aboard the train, I read:

I must start by saying that I am immensely proud of Carl in completing this book. It took a great deal of courage. Well done! It has given us the opportunity for a miracle.

Writing this contribution has been a real struggle for me. Where to start? The biggest tests I have experienced so far in my life have been coming to terms with my own childhood, years of depression and the end of my thirty-year marriage. So when I read what Carl had written about me – the abuse, the lack of love that he needed, and my call-for-help suicide attempt which engendered his fear of loss and inappropriate attachments – I went straight into attack-and-denial mode, calling him a liar, asking him to withdraw his account and wanting no part in it (I was word-processing his handwritten manuscript at the time). It has tested my image of myself as a wife and mother. Aidan will probably never need to write his story, but I thank him for his insight into our family dynamic.

My initial shock and protests were replaced by tearful discussions and truth-telling and I have accepted that this is his version of our lives: there is no absolute truth. But our story as told here will hopefully help parents and children who read it to be completely honest with each other, and to respect one another. After this experience our relationship will withstand any challenge life may present to us.

I was un-maternal but I have grown into motherhood and I now understand what it is all about. To maintain good relationships with our children we need to continually re-evaluate them, and they us as they mature. Talk to them; learn to respect them; let them make their own mistakes without judgement; be there for them. It's a lifelong learning process, but there's no better investment.

My ability to accept this book is mainly due to where I am in my life – several years into a spiritual journey that started with 'The Road Less Travelled', and now centres on a personal relationship with God that gives me the strength to deal with any situation life throws at me, that has helped me conquer the demon of depression.

I love you both so much, my wise sons. You are my best teachers.

I texted her

'Love you so much too. Thanks Mom XXX'

15

'From here to eternity, with love...'

'From Here to Eternity' Giorgio Moroder

It was that sagacious philosopher Fergie – Sarah Ferguson, not the Black Eyed Pea – who I first heard, guesting on *Oprah* I think, utter the idiom:

> *'The past is history,*
> *the future is a mystery,*
> *the present is a gift.'*

It may be feasible that Fergie had lifted it from some self-help epistle she'd read whilst sat under a blue plastic pyramid or having her toes sucked; or that she was paraphrasing a near-identical line from an Eleanor Roosevelt poem; but as Oogway, the turtle in the movie *'Kung Fu Panda'*, said it too, I'd wager it was him whom Fergie was quoting.

But the present truly is a gift.

In recent months I *finally* got to pogo front-row at a Toyah gig; I did a photo-shoot with Marc Almond and, now that we're both clean of addiction we shared nothing stronger than a fruitcake and a pot of chamomile tea; I went to see Marc Almond in concert at the Royal Festival Hall performing

'*Torment & Toreros*' in its entirety, and could enjoy it for the sublime masterpiece it is without being crippled by teenage insecurity; I bid highest on a Siouxsie photograph in a charity auction, and had her sign it, '*To Carl, Fuck off & get your night bus home, love Siouxsie Sioux X*'; and Mom, clearing out her attic, found a photo album of mine from the '80s...

'*Embrace that inner child,*' my hypnotherapist once advised – and that includes my teenage self. Now, looking at those old photos, I'm as fiercely proud of him – both for his sheer artistry and for the balls he had to walk the streets dressed like the love child of Boy George and Marie Antoinette – as I am of Mom.

We only cry from laughing nowadays.

"Why would anyone wanna put themself through *that*?" she asks as we're watching a documentary on gender re-assignment.

"Imagine if y*ou'd* been born in the wrong body, if *you'd* been born with a knob," I say.

"Well it'd save me chasing after it," she larks, that soul mate still eluding her – although not for want of putting herself about: personal ads, toy-boys, S&M soirées, you name it...

"Yeah, *you* use *TENA Lady* to mop up seminal fluid, not because your bladder's going," I rib.

"If I ever get Alzheimer's, put a pillow over my head," she says, as we remember Nan on the eighth anniversary of her death.

I grab a cushion, leap the width of my living-room and, compressing it on her face, I josh,

"Let's take out some insurance!"

"Stop it! I'm gonna wet myself," she laughs, tickling me to deactivate me, the two of us disintegrating in fits of laughter and floundering around on the parquet like two overgrown toddlers.

I tell her, "I'm taking you to a nice little clinic in Geneva tomorrow!

★★★★

After two months of interminable downpour, today Apollo has come up trumps, mercury scheduled to bust thirty degrees later. It's incredible that my indiscreet gob and Mom's intrinsic nosiness didn't scupper the surprise, but I get her to the Eurostar departure gate and across Paris without spoiling it.

An open-top cornflower-blue Renault 2CV awaits us at the steps of Palais Garnier, the grandiose opera house. Okay, it's not quite the chauffeured cabriolet I'd wanted to hire. *You* try sourcing one – weeks trawling the internet, petitions on Facebook and Twitter, telling Mom *Don't go on Facebook 'til further notice* – it's impossible; and it's twenty-eight years since I drove, so reacquainting myself on hectic Parisian boulevards in a left-drive rental car is a non-starter – but like Marianne Faithfull's ex Mick sings:

> 'You can't always get what you want,
> but if you try sometimes,
> you might just find,
> you get what you need.'

I introduce us to the driver; she responds in broken English, "Allo, bonjour; ah am Lucy." Of all the girls' names and of all the tourists she could've driven today!

I recount the song's lyrics, and tell Lucy – sturdy of

forearm and steely of eye and the sort of monsieur no drivers are likely to cut up – "Drive us anywhere, but drive fast!"

Mindless of heat-beaten pedestrians indolently crossing roads, Lucy races down Avenue de l'Opéra, down Rue de Rivoli, past the Centre Georges Pompidou...

With the warm wind in her hair, in her early seventies, only thirty-four years behind schedule, 'The Ballad of Lucy Jordan' is coming true for Mom, except unlike Lucy Jordan she won't descend into madness by song's end.

Across Pont Marie to the Île Saint-Louis, past Notre Dame and on to Saint-Germain-des-Prés, we are deposited for lunch at Les Deux Magots – the historical watering-hole of the literary elite where, in the ivory panelling and Doric pilasters and mosaic floors, and varnish-sealed into the mahogany furniture, the auras of long-dead Simone de Beauvoir and Jean-Paul Sarte are still palpable.

"What a perfect day it's been," trills Mom as we promenade past the Pyramide du Louvre. En route to the Gare du Nord I spot that her right hold-up stocking has slithered to below her knee and that one of her substantial stick-on shoulder pads has absconded so she has developed a foam bicep. As she repairs herself I chide,

"I've got one word to say to you: *Dignitas!*"

and we laugh and laugh and laugh...

★★★★

I pray it will be a long, long way away 'til her time is up. And she's so gregarious, so beloved that I know there will be hundreds at her funeral who I've never met. But nobody will need to ask, *'So, who are you?'* because anyone can tell I am my mother's son. And thank God. Because although hers was tough love sometimes – and there are things I'd have done no differently had I teetered a mile in her stilettos *and* with a son like I was – she made me who I am.

She is the best friend I'll ever have.

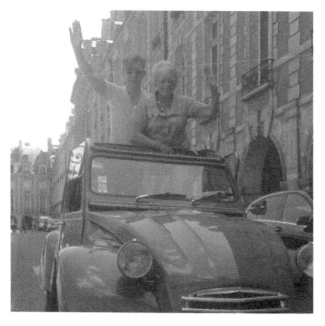

Mom and me in Paris

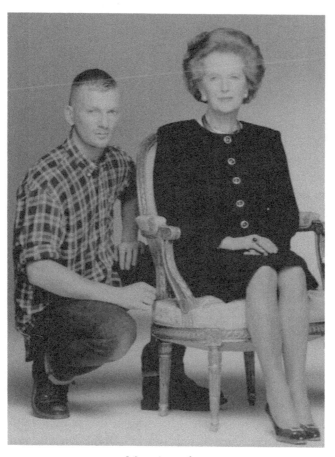

Maggie and me.
photo: Fergus Greer

bonus chapter
'You're history...'
Shakespear's Sister

Today was a scorcher, the hottest day since the heatwave of '76. I'd taken reprieve under the canopy of Compton's Café in London's gay village, sipping my drink to wring maximum value from its over-inflated price, chain-smoking Gitanes Blondes, oozing Chanel elegance in my houndstooth check jacket and chunky gold chain necklaces and black velvet Capri pants and loafers...

The skimpiest winter ray of sun was enough to induce one or two Adonises to strut Old Compton Street shirtless, so this afternoon they were out in force. With their biceps and pecs the size of cannonballs, their twelve-packs – and muscles I didn't even know existed before emigrating to London, much less the names of – I'd christened them the Grade A's. I'd baptised those with hand-grenade-sized biceps, pecs, and six-packs Grade B's. Next in the pecking order were the Grade C's, and those who didn't pump iron were 'D's, but only the svelte ones. The tubby ones I had tagged 'U' for 'undesirable', as tubbies were lepers on this meat market. Birmingham's homo-superior had barely evolved to lower 'C', but even they had been few and far between. Nor did Birmingham's gay scene have a dress code: Man at C&A *Miami Vice* suits, snow-washed denim, anything went. But down here, whether 'A',

'B', 'C' or 'D', the G.I. – gay issue – was combats or blue jeans, length immaterial. Almost all sported buzz cuts, although I'd detected that Mohawks or Nick Kamen DAs didn't ruffle feathers. Long hair, however, was a non grata. I'd seen queers from all four strata overtly sneer at the handsomest long-haired 'A'. Provided his hair wasn't long, 'A' reigned supreme by dint of buffness, not handsomeness, and 'A's had carte blanche to procure their prey at will....

Some ug-mug 'A' who'd cocked a rearward glance to re-examine whoever had sparked his libido had made a U-turn, and in seconds, without a gentleman's excuse-me, was tongue-raping some Depp-faced 'D'; they unlocked lips, and after a brief exchange off they trolled, Ug's hand down the back of Depp's 'fuck-me' Daisy Dukes...

If copping off's that easy, why can't I? I lamented, sipping my café frappé through a straw.

Deep-down, I did know why though: I just couldn't confess it to myself quite yet...

At that moment the catcalls began:
"HILDA OGDEN!"
"MRS MANGLE!"
"NORA BATTY!"

I didn't need to see her to know it was the moth-eaten tranny I had seen every time I'd come here, because the taunts were always the same unimaginative clichés, just from new mouths. She must've heard them a million times, but all the times I'd seen her I hadn't once heard her bite. *She must be immune to it,* I thought as she trundled past in her regular attire of flowery housecoat, headscarf over rollers, wrinkled tights and Dr Scholl's – and as it did each time I saw her, my mind's eye rewound to her Birmingham counterpart, that slipper-shod, wig-in-curlers tranny from The Vic...

Trannies came below 'U's on Old Compton Street. Those with the balls to brave Soho-by-day were companion-less souls, scurrying by heads bowed, or sat in café-shadows, ringside spectators to Compton Street's trivial sports, sports which didn't seem so trivial to those never picked to play...

Some 'A' solicited, "OI! GRANNY! WHADDYA CHARGE FOR BAREBACK?"

"SORRY DEARIE, *THIS* LANDLADY DOESN'T RENT TO DHSS," she rapped to gales of laughter.

Reasserting his supremacy, 'A' inflated his pecs, tensed his twelve-pack and flexed his biceps, his über-macho posturing a reminder to amnesiac laughers that it was *brawn* which most counted, inferior specimens looking him over enviously long after the giggles prompted by Tranny Landlady's putdown had petered out...

I was singing to myself now, an old Soft Cell B-side.
> *'Fun City, Fun City,*
> *to London experience*
> *Fun city, Fun city...'*

I'd catch myself singing it more often the longer I was in London, and lately I'd been singing it incessantly.
> *'I'm all alone*
> *and I'm lost in this city,*
> *Fun City, Fun City,*
> *so this is Fun City...'*

God, here comes that Goth tranny, how can she still wear that coat in this heat?

I saw her regularly. Usually she'd scuttle up and down Old Compton Street like some fugitive terrified of recognition, in perpetual movement as if she hoped *that* would make her inconspicuous – which it never did.

On a compassionate day I'd applaud her, because – for someone so wretchedly introvert she daren't even look up – being a Goth tranny was a heroic lifestyle-choice in an era of Bros and Jason Donovan, the '80s growing evermore conformist 'til it seemed like Punk didn't happen. On a callous day I'd snigger at the comments I overheard as she scampered by. But today was too hot for ceaseless motion in floor-length astrakhan. I watched her claim the last available *al fresco* seat two tables away from me…

Humidity may have bloated to heights it hadn't done in years, but I couldn't take my jacket off – my semi-sheer crêpe chiffon blouse would be see-through with sweat by now. *If I'm sweating in this, she's gotta be dying in that an' it doesn't even look good* I thought, watching her forage busily in her carpet bag to evade derisory stares.

When she pulled out a Walkman and put on headphones, though I could only conjecture it was catty comments that'd driven her to do that, my pitiless mind decried *She deserves it. She wants to hear what they're sayin', not block it out…*

"That tranny with the black bob thinks she's Shakespear's Sister," I overheard a 'C' say to his two mates.

Fuck you. I'm not a fucking tranny, I wear flat shoes, I thought.

"More like *Shakespear's Blister*, she must be boiling in that fake Chanel," said one of the others.

Needful of reassurance, the reassurance I always sought in mirrors, I fumbled in my handbag for my *Paloma Picasso* compact...

"Her face is like a slapped arse, she should get together with that miserable lookin' tranny in the black fur coat." The third designated himself matchmaker. "They could be miserable together."

My reflection didn't fully placate me...

"Shakespear's Blister wants to be careful she doesn't crack her mirror, last thing she needs is seven years bad luck," wisecracked 'C'two...

Perspiration was doing unkind things to my foundation, but it wasn't irreparable...

"What's worse luck than being a tranny?" asked 'C'one.
"Seven more years being a tranny!" quipped 'C'three.

My lipline – which in kinder climes was unparallelled perfection – had feathered, one of my false eyelashes was coming unstuck, but both were rectifiable...

"HILDA OGDEN!" presaged Tranny Landlady's second-coming and diverted me from my reflection...

That'll be that tranny Goth in twenty years...

As she lumbered by, 'C'three prophesied, "That'll be Shakespear's Blister in twenty years!" All three cackling...

Laugh all you wanna, you cunts, that won't be me. I'm not a fucking tranny, I'm a – I returned to my reflection *– a…a…a…*

What the fuck am I?

A New Romantic?

A Gender Bender? A…

I'd been in denial way too long, but suddenly how the world really saw me stared back: I could label myself however I wanted, but to Old Compton Street's collective eye I was no different to that Goth tranny, out of synch with the times, just a ringside spectator sat in café-shadows without friends. And, okay, on my night-time forays to *Kinky Gerlinky, Bang* and *The Daisy Chain,* Boy George, Tasty Tim and Princess Julia might stop to say 'Hi' but in the London clubs I was a ringside spectator too, not outrageous enough to vie with the likes of Leigh Bowery.

Eight lonely, sexless weeks was long enough to realise I wasn't going to make friends, much less get laid, if I carried on dressing like this. Truth be told, I didn't even *want* to dress up anymore: it was just a habit these days, an addiction which – minus the euphoria of the adulation I'd enjoyed in Brummie clubland – had no highs. And most ridiculous of all was, there was an alright man underneath the drag, certainly better-looking than those toxic 'C's who were now misjudging how dire my complexion must be, seeing as I was plastering on more Polyfilla.

I want to walk in the sun, I want to be fancied, I want to strut shirtless through Soho, and if I start lifting weights I could easily be 'C', maybe a 'B', with willpower perhaps even be an 'A', I thought, chucking my compact and foundation in my bag and bolting indoors to the café toilet.

I tore off my jacket, necklaces, earrings and false eyelashes and dumped them behind a U-bend. I wouldn't need them again. I scrubbed my face clean. I'd never wear make-up again, and *not* because of anything derogatory I'd overheard any bitchy queen say today – because over the last six years there wasn't any insult I hadn't heard – but because I'd been there, done that, fought that fight and bought the t-shirt.

And anyway, the bottom line was that I'd moved to London to become a make-up artist, not to waste four hours tarting *myself* up every day. I'd already wasted nearly four years since leaving school doing that whilst finding the time to fail Art College *and* row daily with Mom *and* sign-on every fortnight *and* party so hard that I was never sober long enough to have a hangover....

I wet my hair and slicked it back. I'd go and find a barber straightaway and get my bob cut off, then buy some bleach and a ginger colorant, dye my hair back to its natural colour tonight.

As I left Compton's Café, the Goth tranny looked up at me. I smiled at her. She smiled back. I'd never disdainfully frown at her or any other tranny ever again, because I more than anyone knew the strength of character it takes to tread that path. For me, those cross-dressing, gender-bending, New Romantic '80s were dead.

It was July '89.

I was a blank canvas.
Let London do with me what it would…

To see more photos, or to share your own stories
or thoughts about 'Kiss & Make Up', please
connect with me through Facebook at
'Kiss & Make Up by Carl Stanley'

thanks

★

A huge thank-you to Steve Pottinger for taking a punt and for all your hard work, and to Uli for being a boyfriend above and beyond the call of duty when all I talked about was 'Kiss & Make Up'

Thank-you Marc, Toyah, Lorraine, Neil and Princess Julia for your kind words, Sean Chapman for getting my manuscript to T, and Paul Burston for inviting me to read at Polari before I found a publisher

Thank-you Sarah Fuller for the wonderful cover illustration, and Nicky Johnston for the great photo

Thank-you Linus Pell for the amazing cover design and for three decades of love, laughter, tears and will-they-won't-they

Thank-you Susie Savage for your encouragement to carry on when I couldn't find a publisher

Thank-you Stevo Morgan, David Wright and everyone else who has supported me on Facebook, especially the Birmingham posse, in no particular order: Maggie De Monde, John Lupton, Julie Bedwell, Wayne Evans, Twiggy, Patti Bell, Nick Hynan, Porl and Steve McHale, Dave Lolley, Jan Nolan, Patty Heron, Tracey Aldenhoven, Denise Haddon, Susan Latham, Jason Cooper, Anne Nicholls, Mandy Jane Caldicott, Shannah Jay, Jackie Corrigan, Maz Mulcreevy, Bridget Callaghan, Debbie Ashmore, Cheryl Ann Hardy, Jacki Cottom, Debbie Graves, Lee Jones, Clair Louise Virtue, Bryan Reavenall, Tina Mais, Nicci Fors, Diane Tissington, Mary Whitehouse, Denise Alcott, Cheyenne Mendez, Mark Farrell, Chris Haydn, Maggie Fuzzbox, Neil Blackwell, Laurence Goodridge, Marc Linekar, Janet Dixon, Grace Garvey, Nikki Smith, Jane Tiga Elliot, Lara Ratnaraja, Nadine Hayward, Sian Howarth, Pamela Chapman and anyone who ever went to The Kipper Club, Zig Zag, and Powerhouse on a Wednesday.

To Duncan McCabe, John Monoghan, Martin Hall, Neal Taylor, Wincey, Suman, Esther Anderson and the Thursday night gang. To Lizzie Roleston, Dipika Parmar-Jenkins and Jane Sked who didn't make it into the book because the final edit didn't cover that period. To Veronica for being the first New Romantic I met, and Rae Marie Workman for taking me to the dark side. To Sandra 'Smuffle' Farmer for making me laugh so hard all through junior school and Abigail Chesterton for still being crazy after all these years

Thank-you Chris Barker and Richard James

Thank-you Gary 'Dark Lady' Ahrens for making the mid-'90s one long boozy lunch, and Zoe Manzi for the more-civilized-but-no-less-fun lunches this millennium

Special thanks to David Hodge, Richard 'Sticky Monster' Stockman, Richard Sewell, Andrew Carter, Jason Halsey, Mark Sutherland, Trevor Goodlad, Leonard Hughes, Minty, Mark Tyme, Joe D Ryner and Billie Ray Martin who have had to put up with me not being as good a friend as I should be whilst writing this book, and to Polly Self for being a cantankerous old c★★★ and causing an argument even when there's nothing to argue about

Thank-you Dad, and Aidan and his family

And the biggest THANK-YOU of all to Mom for having the bravery to let me write this book and for seeing the bigger picture.

Carl Stanley

soundtrack

★

Moments Of Pleasure	Kate Bush
Fade To Grey	Visage
Boys Keep Swinging	David Bowie
It's A Mystery	Toyah
Sound Of The Crowd	The Human League
Good Morning Universe (live)	Toyah
Planet Earth	DuranDuran
Pinky Blue (Dance Mix)	Altered Images
Party Fears Two	The Associates
Church Of The Poison Mind	Culture Club
Soul Inside	Soft Cell
Nightshift	Siouxsie and the Banshees
The Crusher	The Cramps
Confusion	New Order
Too Drunk To Fuck	Dead Kennedys
Nipple To The Bottle	Grace Jones
Native Love (Step By Step)	Divine
Kick in the Eye	Bauhaus
Black Heart	Marc and the Mambas
My Little Book of Sorrows	Marc and the Mambas
Between The Lines	Janis Ian
Sex Crime (Nineteen Eighty-Four)	Eurythmics
Victims	Culture Club
No Feelings	Bananarama
Other Voices	The Cure
Fire	The Crazy World of Arthur Brown
Love To Love You Baby	Donna Summer

Love in a Void	Siouxsie and the Banshees
Bring Me the Head	
Of The Preacher Man	Siouxsie and the Banshees
When The Wild Calls	Swans Way
No GDM	Gina X
The Ballad of Lucy Jordan	Marianne Faithfull
You've Lost That Loving Feeling	The Human League
Midnight	Yazoo
Venus In Furs	The Velvet Underground
From The Flagstones	Cocteau Twins
Hall Of Mirrors	Kraftwerk
You Spin Me Round (Like A Record)	
(Performance Mix)	Dead or Alive
The Twist	Klaus Nomi
Rock Lobster	The B-52's
Ignore the Machine	Alien Sex Fiend
Since Yesterday	Strawberry Switchblade
Santa Maria (Wah-Hey Mix)	Tatjana
Runaway (Original Flava 12" Mix)	Nuyorican Soul
Never Lost His Hardcore (Baby Doc Remix)	NRG
Goodbye Yellow Brick Road	Elton John
Power Of Goodbye	Madonna
Falling	Kylie Minogue
From Here To Eternity	Giorgio Moroder
Torment	Marc and the Mambas
Fun City	Marc and the Mambas
You're History	Shakespear's Sister

organisations

★

If you have been affected by any of the issues in
'Kiss & Make Up' and seek professional guidance,
please contact the following organisations:

National Bullying Helpline
Website: www.nationalbullyinghelpline.co.uk
Tel: 0845 22 55 787

Samaritans
Website: www.samaritans.org
Tel: 08457 90 90 90

Alzheimer's Society
Website: www.alzheimers.org.uk
Tel: 020 7423 3500

Narcotics Anonymous
Website: www.ukna.org
Tel: 0300 999 1212

Stonewall – LGB Support
Website: www.stonewall.org.uk
Tel: 0800 050 20 20

PANDAS – Pre and Postnatal
Depression Advice and Support
Website: www.pandasfoundation.org.uk
Tel: 0843 28 98 40

Relate – The Relationship People
Website: www.relate.org.uk
Tel: 0300 100 1234

Wild Thing

This dark, compelling novel from author Joolz Denby is breathtaking in its scope and imagination.

Amnie Wynter has walked away from the glamour of the music industry and gone back north, shedding her old life and re-training as a social worker. Then a brutal killing turns her life upside-down, and Annie has to choose - will she break the rules she lives by?

The decision she makes will change her life forever.

"Denby's hair-raising novel manifests our most primordial fears in an authentic contemporary setting."

The Guardian

Also available from Ignite Books

City Baby

Birmingham punk band GBH are legends within the music scene – gigging and touring continuously for over thirty years, making music, making friends, and making trouble, while never *quite* hitting the big time.

In this candid, hilarious, and moving memoir, their bassist Ross Lomas tells his story. It's the story of how punk rock, and love, saved his life.

'Absolutely captivating'
Vive Le Rock

'Always compelling'
Record Collector

'A fascinating and essential read.'
Louder Than War

Now in its third edition.

Ignite Books is a small, independent publisher.

This book is the latest in our series which we hope puts fresh, thought-provoking, entertaining writing before a new audience. We have a lot of fun doing this, but we also survive on a shoestring budget and a lot of graft. So, if you've enjoyed this book, please tell your friends about us.

You can also find us on Twitter @ignitebooks, so drop by and say hallo. And to learn more about what we do, or shop for our other publications, just visit our website at ignitebooks.co.uk

Thank you.